Bob + Sal[illegible]

SURGEON OF HOPE

BY Jeanette Lockerbie

Tomorrow's at My Door
The Image of Joy
"Just Take It From the Lord, Brother"
The Dino Story (with Dino Kartsonakis)
Fifty Plus
Surgeon of Hope (with Ralph L. Byron, M.D.)

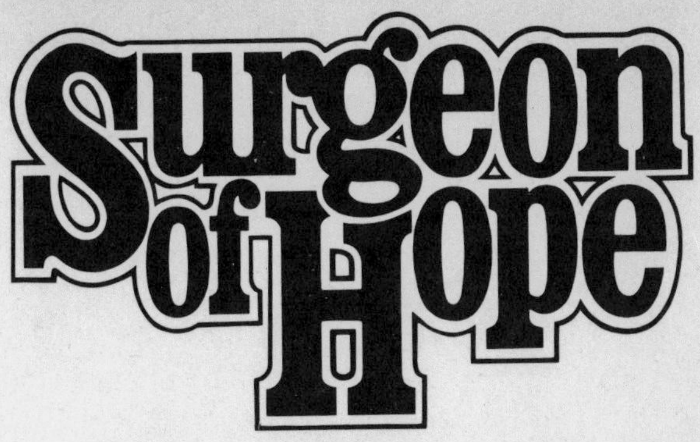

Ralph L. Byron, M.D.
with Jeanette Lockerbie

Fleming H. Revell Company
Old Tappan, New Jersey

Unless otherwise identified, Scripture quotations in this volume are from the King James Version of the Bible.

Scripture quotations identified NIV are from the NEW INTERNATIONAL VERSION. Copyright © 1973 by New York Bible Society International and are used by permission.

Library of Congress Cataloging in Publication Data

Byron, Ralph L
Surgeon of Hope.

1. Byron, Ralph L. 2. Surgeons—California, Southern—Biography. 3. Duarte, Calif. City of Hope. 4. Medicine and Christianity. 5. Congregationalists—California—Pasadena—Biography. I. Lockerbie, Jeanette W., joint author. II. Title.
R154.B98A37 617'.092'4 [B] 76-56742
ISBN 0-8007-0837-7

TO the City of Hope—its ideals of compassionate care for the whole person—its untiring research in the war against catastrophic diseases—and the host of persons whose willing sacrifice makes it all possible.

Acknowledgments

The authors wish to express their gratitude and appreciation: to Aaron Levenstein for his generous permission to reprint excerpts from his book, *Testimony for Man;* to The King's Couples, those who shared from their own experience and the entire class who prayed about this book; to Dr. Raymond C. Ortlund for graciously writing the foreword and showing genuine interest in the book; and to Mr. Dewey Cass whose persistent "You *are* going to do this book?" had much to do with hooking the coauthor.

Contents

Foreword

For seventeen years now my friend Doc and I have been tuned in on the same frequency. What that means is, I stay tuned to *his* frequency.

When I came that long ago to my present pastorate, the Lake Avenue Congregational Church in Pasadena, Doc was doing his typical dead-run thing—teaching a large, successful Sunday school class at the First Presbyterian Church of Hollywood, then bolting over the freeway to Pasadena to teach a large, successful Sunday school class at our church a half hour later! Since his membership was with us, he eventually gave up the Hollywood class, but is still teaching the same Sunday school, the King's Couples, class at Lake Avenue. My friend Ralph is a man born running.

He moves. At the famous City of Hope Hospital where he is chief surgeon, he really covers the place. Then when working hours are over, it's nothing for him to drive three hours to speak to a Bible class or an evangelistic outreach group somewhere.

Get to know Doc Byron. Note his compassion: he cares with medical expertise.

Observe his integrity: you can depend on finding him close to where you last saw him.

See his commitment: he's a kneeling Christian. Learn from him at this point, and you'll never be the same.

But don't dismiss him as a *spiritual giant*—whatever that means—with connotations of being unreal. Ralph Byron bleeds and stumbles and laughs and gets embarrassed, too.

Through the eyes of another dear friend and Lake Avenue member, Jeanette Lockerbie, you have a chance to get to know this remarkable, gifted man. Take it. He is truly a surgeon of hope!

RAYMOND C. ORTLUND, D.D.

Preface

Nothing was more unlikely than that Ralph Byron would one day write *M.D.* after his name—his mother spent years brainwashing him away from his father's profession.

It was equally unlikely that *Bible teacher* would ever apply to him—at an early age he was prejudiced towards Christians as being too satisfied with the mediocre, while to him the pursuit of excellence was everything.

Surgeon of Hope is the tale of how these improbabilities became living fact.

I had heard of Dr. Byron before I met him. His position as chief of surgery at the world-renowned City of Hope spoke for his professional achievement. But this was never the primary focus of talk about him, I noticed. Rather it was Dr. Byron the guest speaker at Christian functions, the Bible lecturer, the teacher of an impressive Sunday school class, King's Couples—and always there was reference to his phenomenal knowledge of the Bible and his ability to quote it verbatim (as though he had cornered the market). People seemed to remember his sayings, and they quoted him: "God always accepts a person at his own level of commitment" and "What we think is ultimately lived out in our lives" and other such memorable thought provokers. The saying that stuck in my own mind the first time I heard him (at a college commencement) was related to his own field of cancer surgery: it revealed his concern for the person, not the *disease,* as he stated, "The ultimate fear of the cancer patient is that at some point we will abandon him," and he went on to explain the reassuring measures that alleviate such fear.

In the course of working on the book, I attended Dr. Byron's King's Couples class and learned what makes his teaching unique; I shared in their fun times that are such a part of the class outreach program, and was impressed with the consistent Christ-centeredness of it all.

Becoming acquainted with the City of Hope through Dr. Byron's eyes was a once-in-a-lifetime experience as together we tramped the beautiful grounds and ins and outs of buildings, some which house fantastically costly modern equipment that spells HOPE for the victims of catastrophic diseases. With unpracticed eyes I viewed the lab areas and marveled at the importance of the humble fruit fly to research. The nearest I got to surgery was trying on a pair of surgical booties at the thus-far-and-no-farther swinging door. The beautifully appointed children's wing brought a lump to my throat as Dr. Byron explained how the playthings are such as *little people who bruise easily* (victims of leukemia) can safely enjoy. We walked through the famous rose garden with its very special City of Hope rose.

I observed the friendly physician in an interchange with a recovering patient: "My daughter brought these flowers for you, Doctor. I grew them myself," the patient managed to say through a maze of tubes. In a hallway we were intercepted by the staff huddling over something. "Here's Dr. Byron, let's ask him." Together we dodged a white-coated man with a telltale *red cart* (cobalt). It's a hospital, it's a center of scientific research, but everywhere we went I sensed that indefinable something that *is* the City of Hope.

The book begins before the City of Hope years, however. As a young man Ralph Byron promised God he would be His man "standing in the gap." This vow has permeated and directed his life to this day. As a U.S. Marine Corps doctor, it troubled him that the troops were going into battle and many of them didn't know Christ as Savior. The chaplain's edict, "You will *never* hold evangelistic meetings as long as I am chaplain," was just a challenge to be met. Even the threat of court-martial did not stop Byron. He never permitted obstacles to deter him. Where there were opportunities, he took them; when there were none, he made things happen.

Basically a rather shy man, Dr. Byron nevertheless bends in every direction to help people, to literally bear the other person's burden. This penchant has taken him into a number of unlikely ventures as he has bailed Christians out of a hole. For instance, one such case of helping involved him with a race car driver.

If (as is true of some in the medical profession) there appears to be an unconscious bid for omnipotence in all this helping hand, with Dr. Byron in its outworking, everyone around him is benefited, materially and spiritually. Nor is anyone left in any doubt as to the source of any *greatness* he might have: "I am what I am by the grace of God" is a life maxim with this doctor.

He's a family man. Next to Jesus Christ, without a doubt, the *little corporal* (his wife, Dorothy) is tops in his life. To spend time with the Byron family is to be assured a lively if not a *hilarious* time! They laugh with and at each other, no one becoming more convulsed than Dr. Byron himself.

The overriding theme of *Surgeon of Hope* is that God does take a man at his own level of commitment—that in the outworking of His plan for this man's life, God moves in everyday affairs—He ploughs something of the miraculous into the man's life, and ultimately brings him to the place of divine appointment. For Dr. Ralph Byron this place is the City of Hope.

JEANETTE LOCKERBIE

SURGEON OF HOPE

1 Finding a Better Way

I untied the surgical mask, peeled off the gloves, and stepped out of my gown. The smile playing on my still sweaty face was a good omen to the anxiously waiting family as I approached them.

It had been a tricky bit of surgery, and the outcome gave me a good feeling. I was thanking God for the excellent team I had working with me. I was grateful, too, for our improved techniques in this particular operation, a bilateral adrenalectomy.

In 1951 Charles Brenton Huggins, a professor of urologic surgery at the University of Chicago Medical School, reported that the removal of the adrenal glands was helpful in certain patients with advanced breast cancer. (The adrenals are small glands the size of a half-dollar which lie near the superior pole of each kidney. Among other things they produce cortisone, adrenaline, and certain other hormones. Since cortisone is essential for life, if the glands are removed, one must take cortisone for the rest of his life.)

As we repeatedly performed this operation, however, a tragic cloud hung over each surgery, a 15 percent mortality rate (approximately one patient in seven died!). But, as Thomas Edison said, "There is a way to do it better; find it." Certainly this is true in surgery. If an operation is carrying with it a high mortality or poor results, then it's important to find this better way, to see if by modifying or changing the surgery, the problems can be solved. In this instance we made two changes in our attempts to solve the problem. We approached the adrenals from the front instead of the back, and reversed the order of their removal. The gratifying result was a drop in the mortality rate to 4 percent (one in twenty-five) which is acceptable in such a major operation.

No patient is just a *case* at the City of Hope. No surgery is *routine.* Nor does my personal philosophy of humanity made in the image of God permit me to be less than highly interested in each of my patients. I had approached this surgery as I do all the others.

The patient is briefed in advance and allowed to ask any questions which unanswered might cause misunderstanding or apprehension which we can help to clear up. Knowing the tendency for patients to hear but not comprehend, my usual practice is to have them tell back to me what I have explained.

Just as important is my personal preparation. In my early morning appointment with God, I spend time praying for my work and my particular surgery of the day. By the time the operation is to begin, I am prepared.

I walk through the *No Admittance* doors to the operating suites, don *booties* (covers for my shoes), change into a scrub suit, put on a disposable hat and mask, and then, as do my assistants, I scrub my hands and arms for ten minutes. Hands held up so the water drips off the elbows, I back through the swinging doors into the operating room proper. The scrub nurse has preceded me and now helps me put on my sterile gown and gloves. The battle to prolong life is on. As a team, we go into action.

The area for surgery, in this case the abdomen, is cleansed and painted with antiseptic solution; sterile drapes are positioned, and the suction and cautery are connected. An incision is made on the right side first so the abdomen may be explored to determine if the surgery is technically possible. Once the operability is established, the incision is completed.

Traditionally, operating rooms are emotion packed, characterized by rough language, excited bursts of anger directed at an assistant or the hapless scrub nurse, and a dramatic tenseness. The emotional outbursts are generally excused because of the seriousness of the situation—*a life is hanging in the balance.* The Lord has taught me, however, that one doesn't have to flare up with temper or harsh words. In the operating room, as elsewhere, it is possible to be relaxed and to display the deep-seated peace which

God has given. I don't get angry—and I find that my assistants don't either. Not all surgeons act alike. I carry on a running conversation, explaining the surgery, pointing out anatomical landmarks, and yes, sometimes sharing humorous incidents in similar operations. An onlooker's first impression might be that a sloppy job is being done. Nothing is further from the truth.

I approach the right adrenal, the more difficult, first. It lies against the vena cava under the liver. One misplaced cut—and the hemorrhage is unbelievable. When working in such a cavity, gentleness is the order of the day, as it is in all surgery. It's during the dissection of the right adrenal that I am in great danger of getting into trouble with bleeding. The rule when I'm in difficulty is a simple one: Everyone gets into trouble; it's the good surgeon who knows how to get out.

Right and then left adrenal removed, I check for bleeding. There is none. I close up the abdomen, remove the drapes, and get out of my gown. Only then am I conscious of how hard I've been working and that I am perspiring. How true it is what a surgeon at the turn of the century said:

> No one knows the haunting anxiety, the deep sense of responsibility, and the numerous self-reproaches of the man who spends his life as an operating room surgeon. He must have a hand as light as floating perfume, an eye as quick as a darting sunbeam, a heart as compassionate as all humanity, and a soul as pure as the waters of Lebanon!

The surgery over, I pull on a pair of overalls, and go to see the relatives of the patient. As I approach, their eyes are riveted on my face; they're searching for a telltale expression that will indicate success or failure. My satisfied smile is their answer. A smile is a curve that can straighten out many things. This is never more true than when a positive postoperative verdict is given by the doctor. I give the relatives a brief description of the surgery.

Built into big cancer surgery is the fact that the patient is often in poor condition to start with; he is frightened, worried, and frequently feels very weak. His morale may be at a very low ebb. To take such a patient successfully through a five- or six-hour operation is difficult at best, nor is there consolation in losing such a patient, and trying to justify the failure by his poor condition. There is no easy way to lose, so it's always especially rewarding when I'm able to assure the loved ones as well as the patient, that the surgery is successful. I breathe a thank-you to the Lord.

A brief respite before my next assignment gives me time for reflection on how vastly satisfying is my life here at the City of Hope, this oasis in the desert, this mecca for the victim of a catastrophic disease. My mind turns to the near miracles that brought me here more than twenty years ago, the unpredictables God has ploughed into my life, and His pinpoint timing that kept me on a step-by-step course, as He prepared me for the work He had planned for me.

With a glance at my watch I stride back toward the operating area pondering how I might so easily have missed out on all of it, how I might have become almost anything *but* a doctor!

My father was a doctor, a general practitioner, and as long as I can remember, my mother was on a crusade to push me as far as she could away from medicine. As I reached my teens the dialog would go something like this:

"What do you think you would like to do with your life, Ralph?" Mother would ask. I would give a casual answer, "Oh, I don't really know, Mother. Maybe I'll become a lawyer, and I've thought about politics, or a teaching career."

"One thing you don't want to go into is medicine," Mom would counter.

Though I was pretty sure what her answer would be, from previous discussions on the subject, I would say, "Why not? What's wrong with medicine. *Dad's* a doctor."

"That's just it," Mother would retort. "You know how hard your father has to work—all the night calls—your life's just not your own when you're a doctor."

"But," I would suggest, "won't I have to work hard no matter what field I choose?"

"Perhaps you would. But think—your father is just killing himself working so hard, or at least, he's shortening his life."

So, if my mother had any say in the matter, for me medicine was out.

My father's reaction was different. He simply said, "Go into whatever you feel you want to do. Make up your own mind, Ralph. I will support you as long as you're in school." In retrospect, I sense that Dad really wanted me to go into medicine, as he had done, but he carefully concealed this desire. Knowing from experience the price there is to pay, he realized it could be a disaster were he to coerce me into medicine. He wanted any such idea to originate with me, to be my own decision. In this he was very, very wise. Later, when I was struggling in medical school, I knew *I* had chosen this path.

I do not want to give the impression that this was a case of parents arbitrarily pulling in different directions. No, indeed. Rather, they were thinking of what was best for me. I was the only child in the family, so whatever their parental hopes and dreams, they were centered in me. Mother wanted her son to have a life of his own; Dad, although he did not express it at the time, had in mind the long years of training, the grueling demands of hours of study, and the almost superhuman effort that goes into the making of a surgeon. A surgeon fights his way up the ladder in school, struggles to get into medical school, and drives himself relentlessly, pushing toward the pursuit of excellence required for becoming a well-trained doctor. Dad knew the great motivation needed to survive the prolonged ordeal and to achieve the goal; and that through all the rigors of training, the aspiring doctor must never lose his concern for the sick and his compassion for those in need.

Let it be your own decision, Dad counseled.

Anything but medicine, Mother cautioned.

Meanwhile, I had my own half-baked ambitions, football, for one. Then, living as we did in Los Angeles, Hollywood was just a half hour away. The Hollywood of the stars, as it was in those days, lured me, causing me to fancy myself as an actor.

Not yet did I know the One who would take over my ship, who would become the Captain of my soul, and who would wonderfully direct me into finding not just a better, but *the best* way for my life.

2 The City of Hope—What Is It?

The year was 1912. Migration from eastern to western United States was burgeoning. Not all were in search of gold. It was the era of the *white plague* (tuberculosis). Among the migrants seeking life and health in California's hospitable climate, a young Jewish man, coughing and choking on the streets of Los Angeles, found *death.*

In a sense this young man's untimely death might be likened to the analogy Jesus gave of the seed of wheat that fell to the ground and died. For it was from this snuffed out life that a new hope for thousands of victims of the killer disease was kindled.

A handful of concerned Jewish men and women were not content to merely shake their heads and mourn. They decided it was in their power to do something. There was something dauntless about that group—like their father, Abraham.

The need was urgent; the time was short. Other people were dying. Thirty-five men and women, called together by Boris Flatte and Bernard Cohen, formed The National Jewish Consumptive Organization, with Cohen as president. A nine-member committee was appointed. To do what—with what? Their only *assets* were patients.

Their first fund raising effort netted the group $136.05. Only $136.05 to establish a sanatorium! Heady over their desperately needed project, they formulated a constitution and bylaws, with the aid of volunteer young lawyers. In their wildest imagination could the three, Chaim Shapiro, Elias Rosenkranz, and J. Allen Frankel, know their names were to appear again and again in the public activities and minutes of the City of Hope? The prospect was brightening. The next function, a theater party, put $2,400 into the coffers.

In the nearby San Gabriel Valley—once a river bed and at that time a stony, scrubby desert—land was cheap. The $2,400 was the down payment on ten of its arid acres; the total price was five thousand dollars. Two tents comprised the original facilities of the City of Hope.

An author, Aaron Levenstein, saw, admired, and became so interested in the City of Hope that he publicized it in a book, *Testimony for Man*. Of the original site, Levenstein wrote:

> The sun shone brightly on January 11, 1913, when "the committee" journeyed to Duarte, twenty miles from Los Angeles, to open the hospital. The sand crunched under their heels as they raised two tents . . . The drab canvas blended with the sweep of the desert, as if to provide a protective coloration that death might pass by unseeing.

Two tents. Two patients and one nurse. An unimpressive beginning, except, as Isadore Familian, the first vice-president of the organization takes great satisfaction in quoting from the Talmud, "He who has saved one life, it is as if he has saved the whole world."

If the City of Hope were just one more medical facility in the nation, it would still be worthy of our time to note its beginnings, for we will never have enough hospitals. The City of Hope is uniquely worth one's interest, however. Those who pioneered it were proud men. Many were immigrants from the ghettos of Eastern Europe, and they had their own concepts of the dignity of the individual. While it is true that in all the years since those two tents were erected in the desert no patient has ever received a bill from the City of Hope, neither has one patient ever been robbed of his humanity by being made to feel he was a charity case. There's a saying in the Talmud, "Who gives the poor money is blessed sixfold; who gives him morale is blessed sevenfold." Charity can demoralize.

The hard-headed businessman is at a loss to explain how a costly operation such as the City of Hope has survived; not only so, it has steadily expanded.

There were near nightmare years as far as funds were concerned. The depression years took their toll as even the most reliable contributors found themselves in dire financial straits. There were times when the nurses, unpaid themselves for six months, fought back the tears as they worked. The tears were not for themselves, but for the fate of their patients should they have to be sent home because of the lack of funds.

Money is and likely will always be a concern. The City of Hope by deliberate design, operates on the policy that what *must* be done, *should* be done; the raising of the money will follow. It is a radical policy that would destroy any venture except one founded on hope and faith.

No landscape contractors could be hired to beautify the scrubby acreage. But here too, people had a heart. On weekends members of the Los Angeles Junk Peddlers Association drove their wagons to Duarte to contribute odd items that would help to improve the appearance of the grounds. Old-timers in Los Angeles still reminisce of the days when they were children and would visit Duarte with their parents to bring a wagonload of topsoil, to transplant a bush, or to help prepare the parched soil for grass.

The care of the sick historically has been a ministry of religious, compassionate people. Many hospitals still have ties—some looser than others—with a denomination.

The City of Hope, likewise, began as a sectarian undertaking, but was always open to people of all faiths. From its very founding, it could say in the words of Louis Pasteur:

> We do not ask of an unfortunate, what country do you come from, or what is your religion?

We say to him:

> You suffer; that is enough. You belong to us, we shall make you well.

The idea of a medical facility that makes its resources available without any charge has excited Americans of all kinds. Business executives and labor leaders, lawyers and Hollywood actors, college professors and artists, writers and ministers, and government officials and shopkeepers, have all joined forces to expand the City of Hope into a world-renowned center for treatment and research. It is difficult to think of any other enterprise that has won such diversity of support and that has established itself so firmly as a focal point of national unity.

Among the auxiliary workers for the City of Hope, as among its staff, can be found the whole spectrum of political viewpoints. But all suspend their differences in the recognition that the care of the sick is beyond party and beyond political consideration. From the White House, five presidents of the United States from Franklin D. Roosevelt to John F. Kennedy, have hailed the successes of the City of Hope.

What is it, more than so many other hospitals, that has attracted such fervent support? Why is its *character* so vital a theme to so many people?

Very early in its history the founders and builders became aware that their venture involved more than hospital walls and laboratory centrifuges. It was their conviction that the work they were doing was not only useful in itself but had an even more profound meaning than the necessary act of healing. As quoted in *Testimony for Man,* a former president of the City of Hope, the late Seymour Graff stated:

> Finer materials than brick and mortar have gone into this Medical Center. The substance of which it is built is man's humanity to man.

When asked what he considered the most significant aspect of the City of Hope, Judge Bernard S. Selber, of the Los Angeles Superior Court, replied:

> The fact that it not only prolongs the years of life but makes those years better and richer.

If mankind has learned anything from its long history of suffering, it is that no line can be drawn between the material and the spiritual. Whoever divorces the one from the other denies the fullness of life. Our age recognizes the unity of body and soul, but, in practice, interprets this to mean that soul does not exist. The extraordinary *success* of the City of Hope (though *success* needs to be redefined in this context) is proof that our age is not as brittle as it pretends to be. Men do respond—when the right voice calls.

Few of the pioneers whose dreams and hopes and dedication had brought this place into being lived to see tuberculosis brought under control through the dramatic breakthroughs of the fifties and sixties. Yet their concept that every human being, just by virtue of being born, is entitled to the best that science has to offer, regardless of his color, creed, origin, or economic condition, grew more meaningful with the years.

3 Detours and Direction

I have long been convinced that God has a blueprint, a plan, and a purpose for our lives when we commit our way unto Him.

In my own life it was a circuitous route from Los Angeles where I was born, to where God ultimately wanted to use me—a place not more than twenty-five miles from my birthplace.

Looking back from this vantage point we might be tempted to question, since this is obviously where God wanted me, why did He bring me over so many detours? Wouldn't it have made more sense to lead me to this place years earlier? Had I been able to read my future, I possibly would have given God an argument such as, isn't there a shorter route?

A backward look (with the infinite wisdom of hindsight) clearly demonstrates to me that the seeming detours were, in fact, God's direct route for me. Each experience, each *coincidence* (what's a Christian doing with such a word in his vocabulary?), each delay, disappointment, or fortuitous circumstance was a precise part of God's blueprint for my life. I can retrace, in retrospect, each step which led to the next. Even more important, I can perceive the lessons God had to teach me. And at the heart of these lessons are the varied pieces of life that have combined to make me what I am today.

It thrills me that the City of Hope which was to become in reality my theater of operation, had its beginnings about the same time I did. This ties into my basic philosophy that not only does God have a plan but that there is an exact time element to it. I truly believe that God was preparing me for this place, and at the same time He was preparing a place for me to serve Him as I served suffering men and women.

Although hospitals were to play such a major role in my future, unlike the bulk of Americans, I did not first open my eyes in a hospital room. There was a frightful downpour (unusual in Southern California) on that February day, and my mother could not make it to the hospital. A quick boil of the water, a rapid transformation of the bedroom into a delivery room, and I came into the world. A most unimpressive beginning!

My dedicated doctor father was out making his house calls. Could it be that this was the beginning of my mother's determination that her son would be anything but a medical doctor?

I grew up in an old house in an area of Los Angeles that would soon be classed as a slum area. Ours was an adequate house and it was kept in a good state of repair with our postage stamp backyard transformed, in turn, into a baseball diamond, the basketball court, track, and gym.

My early years were uneventful, and very happy. If, as the psychologists tell us, children are affected for life by their childhood relationship with their parents, then I am most fortunate. Mother and Dad loved each other and they loved me and showed it. We did many things together, and without realizing it, I was learning and absorbing lessons they had learned.

Dad had a simple rule: "If a subject is hard for you in school, work a little harder, and it will become easy for you and your favorite subject." Somehow he had picked up and internalized the Winston Churchill maxim: "Never quit. Never, never, never."

School was not too hard for me (maybe because Dad's philosophy kept rubbing off on me). Both parents made studying a game —and I loved games. They had me reading and doing arithmetic even before I got to school.

Though ours was an old neighborhood and the schools were old, the quality of teachers more than made up for any defects in the facilities. Those teachers were dedicated and competent; they were just great to me, and I owe much to them. Also, my mother would frequently do my homework simultaneously with me. Thus, she shared her study patterns with me, helped me if I got stuck, and made sure I did all my assignments. I couldn't know in those early days, the riches that were mine because of such good beginnings in my education. Through years and years of study (that still continues) I have appreciated my teachers and my parents' contribution.

Big doors swing on small hinges. So, in our lives, long range results can stem from seemingly trivial occurrences. As happens with small boys, a new interest threw a monkey wrench into my second grade studies. I fell madly in love with a girl in my class! To remove this distraction to my work, a parent-teacher conference was called which prompted my transfer to a higher grade. From that time on and all through grade and high school, since I was not destined to be very tall, I was always the smallest or next to the smallest in gym class.

My ambition to be a great football player was thwarted. I was simply too short, too small for the game. In retrospect it is apparent that, all unknown to me, God was keeping me on course.

I entered my teens—healthy, enthusiastic, and successful in my schooling. The routine of living, learning, and playing was going well. Somehow, God was not in the picture.

My mother was a Christian who concentrated her involvement to Sunday morning church service and a large adult Bible class which she served as president for a time. She must have believed strongly in prayer for she was the one called by the members of that class when there was a special need for prayer. It was she who made sure I got to Sunday school every week. My regular attendance, however, did nothing to enlighten me as to what vital Christianity is all about. Unfortunately, the Gospel was so veiled that its message simply didn't register with me. Strange as it may seem, though, looking back to those classes I realize that I was always on the side of believing the Bible when the point was argued. It seemed I was a fundamentalist and I wasn't even a Christian!

My father did not profess any religion. He tolerated church activities as long as they were limited to Sunday morning. He was a man of great honesty and integrity; he had a sense of fair play and a willingness to work hard enough to get the job done—and done well. I've heard it said of my father, "He never loses a friend, he just keeps making new ones." He was indeed a much loved physician who under his somewhat gruff exterior had a real heart for people.

Undoubtedly, Dad's position with regard to Christianity had some effect upon my own interest in pursuing it. A superficial look at me would not have disclosed this truth, but my mind was even then cluttered with evil thoughts and unworthy motives. I had a tendency to gravitate toward trouble. Somehow I was attracted to the wrong people for friendship.

A degree of interest in church was generated when a new church built in a better area replaced the one in my deteriorating neighborhood. I was encouraged to attend a youth group. Again, as in Sunday school, either the message was unclear, or it didn't register with me. Until—something happened to two of the young fellows who attended the youth group. They had gone off to a conference, and both had been converted. Jim and Bob were the most changed young men I had ever seen.

What impressed me and captured my imagination as to the cause, was their changed language: their foul-mouthed speech had undergone a total transformation; it had been replaced with wholesome speech. Secondly, their willingness to join me in somewhat wild adventures had disappeared, and this left me wondering. Also, they showed an inordinate interest in reading the Bible and in praying. They even had a concern for me that I would know Christ as my Savior and share this new experience that was theirs.

My first reaction to all of this was that they were approaching the wrong person. I didn't have a need for the Savior. However, after observing the two of them rather closely for a few days, I concluded that whatever they had, it was real. When I got them alone I asked, "What happened to you two? You sure are different."

"I became a Christian," replied Jim, and Bob echoed heartily, "That's right. Me too. We both became Christians."

"What's *that?*" I pried further. "A Christian! Aren't all Americans Christians?"

"No," was the direct answer. "A Christian is one who has received Jesus Christ as his Savior and Lord."

"What did you do that for?" I probed.

"That's what the Bible says to do," was their ready response, and they began to quote the verse in Romans 10:9, "That if thou shalt confess with thy mouth the Lord Jesus . . . ."

"Wait a bit," I interrupted. "I've read the Bible and I've never seen that verse." (True, I had read the first page of Genesis, and you can be sure I had not seen the verse they were quoting to me.)

Not to be intimidated, they opened their Bible and showed me the verse. I saw I wasn't winning, so I changed my attack. "You've just lifted that verse out of the Bible," I accused them. "That isn't the message of the Bible. Moreover, a text taken out of context becomes a pretext."

We had quite an argument. It almost ended in a fistfight. As I walked home alone I had the smug feeling that I had done well in the debate. But a kind of longing mingled with the smugness. Had I won the skirmish and lost the eternal engagement?

4 *I'll* Be That Man, God

I could not forget, could not get away from the two, Bob and Jim, and their changed lives. The hound of heaven was hot on my trail.

I decided to look into this Christianity in earnest; read the Bible, listen to what was said about it, and come to some conclusion concerning this Jesus of the Bible. The more I read, listened, and observed, the more I became convinced that there was indeed a personal aspect to all of it as my two friends staunchly asserted. Bearing in on me was the conviction that I needed a Savior and that Jesus was God who had moved into history to bear our (my) sin in His own body on the cross.

But against this mounting interest was a strong dissuader. I had two major hang-ups with Christianity. One (which I had determined for myself earlier) was that Christians were inferior or at best, mediocre persons. The church we attended was large. There were many young people, and from what I knew of them, they were not overly bright (or so it seemed to me). They tended to be poor students and lacking in talent. As I came to know their parents, I found that they were unimpressive also.

On occasion a missionary on furlough would speak. I don't know where the church members found them, but they too were dull and left me cold. I concluded in my teenage mind that Christians were those who weren't making it in everyday life; so they sought the seclusion of the church. They needed someone to pat them on the back and not expect too much from them—and the church was willing to do this! It was not for me; I had no interest in being that kind of a person.

My second hang-up was related to the first: I had somehow concluded that the pursuit of excellence was not compatible with being a Christian. Perhaps I had sensed right or wrong that to the Christian, excellence and spirituality were mutually exclusive. Added to that was what a football coach had often said, "Nice guys always lose."

Through the years, I've sadly found that in certain Christian circles some interpret a desire for excellence as a worldly ambition. Yet nothing is further from the truth.

So everything relating to the Bible and Jesus Christ inevitably was sifted through my own bias. Nevertheless, as the days passed, I became more and more unable to disregard the inner voice that insistently told me I must take this Jesus as my Savior.

The struggle climaxed the evening I attended the youth group and a visiting speaker gave the message. I recall neither who he was nor what he said that evening. However, what I do remember vividly is that at the closing prayer he asked if anyone would like to receive the Lord Jesus. I could feel the pounding of my own heart. Minutes went by and with them my opportunity was slipping away. At the last instant I raised my hand to indicate that I wanted to accept this invitation. My gesture went all but unnoticed. But God had worked an instantaneous miracle in my life. From that time on, I've always felt it vitally important to offer my listeners a direct opportunity to make a decision. After all, what good is it to lead a person to a filled table, if we do not then invite him to pull up a chair and partake of the good things!

Immediately on my conversion—for such it was that Sunday evening, not mere emotion or fleeting exuberance—I had the desire to do something for God. The cynicism, the critical attitude I previously had held toward Christians, was gone. I was just eager to be useful to God. But there was no immediate opportunity. I prayed, "Lord, I'm ready to serve You *now*." The church people didn't seem to know what to do with me, this eager new convert with so much enthusiasm.

In a meeting one evening the question was asked, "Does anyone have a testimony?" (I was aware from my attendance at such meetings that this meant a statement relating to one's faith in Christ.) I waited for some of the older Christians to get to their feet. No one did. Again, at the last minute, I rose. My voice was a bit wavery; this was a scary thing to do the first time. But I found myself telling those folk what it had been like for me without Christ, how I had come face to face with His claims, what that encounter had done for me, and how wonderful it had been since I had invited Him into my life. Then I sat down.

There was a strange reaction. After the meeting some of my friends came and said, "At the rate you lost friends tonight, if you go on with that testimony business just one more time, you won't have a friend left! Now, why don't you take our advice and settle for *living* what you believe; *not talking* about it."

With those ringing words of questionable encouragement, Ralph Byron, the enthusiast for Christ, went on the shelf. Hereafter asked, "Are you a Christian?" I would say, "Yes, definitely." Should the questioner add, "Are you doing anything about it?" my answer had to be no.

In spite of the blockage, however, I knew I was on a new road; my life *had* changed. I could not be talked out of that. Neither did I do much to nurture this new life. Oh, I prayed a little—very little, I must admit—and I read something from the Bible each day. Of paramount importance, I had made this monumental discovery: in my own life I was proving that being a Christian did not rob one of his goals! Contrary to my previous impression, I now saw that being a Christian made my goal, the pursuit of excellence, much more of a reality.

Excellence—but in what? What was this goal? Where was life beckoning me? Not into *medicine*. My mother's brainwashing was a powerful factor in my thinking.

What then of a God-designed blueprint?

High school days were over. The slogan, *the college of your choice,* not yet coined would have had little meaning for me anyway. The University of California, Los Angeles, UCLA, was my *choice* because it was cheap; for residents of California just twenty-six dollars a semester. I majored in chemistry and math. I played school like a game; played fair but was ruthless if someone got in my way.

I'm not proud of it as I look back and remember. For example, there was a student (I'll call him Bill; not his real name) who was taking organic chemistry in my class at UCLA. Our position in the laboratory had placed us next to each other. The very nature of our proximity resulted in our sharing information, pooling ignorance, and going over problems together. There was an additional tie: my schedule called for two classes at the same hour, so I would go to my physics class one week and chemistry the next. This meant that I desperately needed to copy the notes of someone who was present at the lectures. Bill was a natural and besides, he took notes well. He was more than cooperative and let me use them.

The moment of the big exam approached. Things that weren't clear to me, I asked Bill to explain. He obliged. The exam came and went, followed by the waiting period till the grades came out. When the results were posted, I got a B+—and Bill failed. As if to rub salt into his wounds, these results were posted where everyone could see them.

I cringe even as I write this, to think how I treated this fellow who had helped me so generously. What did I do? Instead of being the one to console him for his failure, instead of helping him to correct his deficiencies and get back on the track, I dropped him like a bad apple. I was success-oriented; he *failed*. I had no more interest in him. Needless to say, he was treated to a double hurt. And although, because of this ruthless trait in me, I crushed this fellow, I was totally unaware at the time of what this did to him.

God was to bring a very special person into my life, one who was instrumental in helping me deal with some of my deplorable characteristics. But that was not yet.

Throughout history God has used many and varied situations and circumstances to shape a life. In my case it was the challenge of a fellow student, tossed in a spirit of rivalry, that totally redirected my future.

"We can't beat you in chemistry, but come on over to biology and we will beat you," he dared me.

I remember as though it were yesterday. I took the bait and enrolled in a comprehensive zoology class. It was my first taste of anything in biology. To my surprise I liked it. I decided to put medicine on my list of possible careers—at the bottom of my list.

There was no thought in my mind of a destiny God had for me. My teenage decision to accept Jesus Christ as my Savior had been real. But, as I have indicated, there was little encouragement and no outlets for my early enthusiasm it seemed. Without the help and the incentive to grow and mature in my faith, I remained virtually a spiritual infant. My life was that of a typical student, and I certainly was not looking for signs that God was interested in moving into my life to mold and shape it.

I was in the chemistry lab one day when a student dashed in and said, "They're giving some kind of an exam for medical school over in the auditorium." I huffed and puffed my way there in time to take what proved to be a medical aptitude test. Then, looking over the courses I'd taken, I discovered that I had the bare minimum requirements for medical school. *Forget it,* I thought, knowing the stiff competition for admission.

But another piece of the jigsaw puzzle of my life was about to surface. A friend of my father came to visit us, and in the course of conversation he asked (naturally since I am the son of a doctor), "Have you applied to medical school?"

"No," I answered, "I'm going on for a master of science degree in chemistry."

As though he hadn't heard me, he continued with, "Do you have a schedule with the deadline for applying?" I knew I had missed by one week. Even so, this man advised me to go ahead and apply. He went so far as to offer to draft the letter for me, then to forward it to the admissions committee.

It seemed harmless enough so I did as he had asked. I *knew* it wouldn't work. I was late in applying and my background studies would disqualify me.

A week later I was accepted in the Medical School of the University of California of San Francisco.

What should I do? Go ahead as planned with my chemistry? Take this unexpected opportunity at medical school? I decided I'd better take this chance.

In mid-August I started. With so little biology, it was devastating. Every word, it seemed, was a new word. At the end of six weeks I wrote my folks, "For the first time in my life I'm flunking out." Ten weeks went by and it was no better. "I'm worse than when I last wrote," I had to admit to my parents.

Feeling myself on rock bottom, I breathed a feeble prayer, "Lord, You've got to help me out of this failure if You want me to be a doctor." I think this was the first time that in a practical, down-to-earth way I linked God with my future.

How did He answer that cry from the depths?

God brought to my mind ideas for a workable, fruitful study pattern. I can never sufficiently thank Him for this. Adequate as this pattern was to insure my success in school, far, far beyond that benefit has been the long-range influence it has had on my life ever since.

Back to my problem in those early days in medicine. It was not only that, like my classmates, I was confronted with an unbelievable amount of material to learn; it was that what we were hearing, seeing, and reading was information that we needed to *retain* if we were to be even average doctors. I couldn't believe how much the professors could cram into five or six hours of lectures and several hours in the laboratories. At the end of my first day, I was a month behind! The problem was compounded by the deluge of new words. A medical student adds five thousand big words to his vocabulary in the first four months! For the first time in our lives we were asked to stretch to the limit our learning ability. We all sensed this, and in our own little ways, tried different methods.

Some of the students felt the way to learn was to spend hours and hours in the evenings in the dissecting laboratory handling and looking at the structures. Others promoted the idea that the trick is to *understand* the material: "If one understands it, he will remember it." Several advocated reading and rereading the books and notes. (This was no easy job inasmuch as it took three to four hours to read it once.) Then there were the outline boys. They would take their notes from the lectures and information from the books, and make a master set of notes—condensed, accurate, and complete. Another group thought that copying one's lecture notes would drive the information into the computer. All of the methods required hard work and lots of it. It was soon apparent there was no easy way. Fred, one of the students, told me, "I have heard the

Campanile (a landmark on the campus) chime one o'clock every night for four months while I have been studying."

I tried all the methods as did the other students. In the final analysis God gave me patterns which would work for me. They were not easy, but they brought results. The specifications were designed to meet the problems of (1) limited time, (2) new words, (3) understanding, (4) retaining, (5) self-accountability, and (6) staying power.

Puck magazine used to have as its caption, "Don't squander time; that is the thing life is made of."

I found this to be so. With the days totally filled, the potential time to study is limited as to the number of hours, and more particularly, by the number of hours that you can remain fresh enough to function effectively. I stretched my time gradually by adding an hour before dinner and two hours early in the morning (5:00 A.M. to 7:00 A.M.). One has to be quite desperate to do this. Although the length of time is limited by your physical strength, it is possible to improve the quality of the time. I had a terrible habit of letting my mind wander as I read or studied. I had a struggle with this. It was so easy for me to read a page while I was thinking about something else. At the end of the page I would discover that I had no idea what I had read. I attempted to correct this problem and must have failed ten thousand times. However, like a baby learning to walk, I would try again. The Lord gave me no instantaneous victory in this, but little by little, I showed improvement.

New words are a major problem; unless one knows them, he is limited in his comprehension and ability to communicate. With me they did not stick just by hearing them or writing them. I found that I had to give a top priority to learning the new words each day. It was helpful to me to list the new words on one side of a page and the definition on the other. Then I would fold the paper in half and quiz myself from word to definition and from definition to word.

Pectoralis major	Muscle from chest to the arm
Scapula	Shoulder blade
Sternocleidomastoid	Neck muscle to turn head

I would go over the list several times until I could do it perfectly. Then several hours later I would review it again and see if I had retained it. A day later and a week later I would quiz myself. This enabled me, long before exam time, to discover how I was doing. It was interesting to me that as I learned the words, I was on the road to learning the material.

Although understanding in part comes from reading, hearing, and seeing, it is necessary to make a conscious effort to be sure one does understand it. I found that the better students tried to use the things they were learning as much as possible. Every Saturday we went to the football game. While everyone else was watching the intricacies of the game, I would be wondering what muscles the quarterback was using to throw the ball and how they were teaming up together. If a player injured his knee, I would be thinking about the ligaments of the knee and how they worked to stabilize the knee. Much of what we were learning could be used as a conversation piece and it required a measure of understanding to do this successfully. There is no doubt that the more one uses information, the better he understands it, and it is a truism that if one understands something, it is easier to learn.

The object in learning is ultimately to retain the material. As Disraeli said, "The secret of success is constancy to purpose." Whether one has to go over material seven times or seventy times seven, there is a point where it becomes yours. The important thing is, it has become *yours*.

I review for two reasons; it greatly aids in my permanently retaining the information, and it enables me to discover if I am failing to remember the material. If I am not going over it enough while I am learning it, I need to know this, and make corrections quickly. Nothing is worse than to assume I know it, and then later on discover that I don't know it at all. On a scale of ten, the original memorizing is at ten for hardness and effort. However, by repeating it becomes progressively easier, and by the seventh time is about a three for hardness. This means that if I have the hard part behind me, I should be willing to review a few extra times as this is the easy but necessary part to making it stick.

I found there was a limit to how hard I could work or how long without a fatigue factor undermining my effort. If I arrived at class in the morning too tired to listen or take notes, I was defeating myself. Also, I knew that my pace had to be one that I could maintain indefinitely. If I am only going to study hard once, I can if necessary, study all night. However, I certainly cannot make it a steady palatable diet. If I get sick from a too rigorous schedule, I defeat myself and am far worse off than I would have been with a lesser effort.

I was to learn that our memories are our most precious possession: in nothing else are we rich; in nothing else are we poor. Likewise, I would discover how unbelievable are our brains in their function, structure, and complexity.

The average brain is made up of 14 billion cells. Two billion of these are nerve cells; the remainder are supporting cells. The brain is like a miniaturized computer, capable of an infinite variety of uses. It is said that even during final college examinations, we use only about one-half of one percent of its potential. We go to school to load and learn to use our computer. There is some evidence that nothing we see, hear, or experience is lost from this wonderful, *multibillion dollar* computer. Information may slip into the subconscious from where we may not easily retrieve it, but it is there contributing to our total makeup. This suggests that we should be careful of what kind of information we put into our computer.

In all my God-directed programming of my own computer in order to become a successful student, God was preparing me to memorize His Word, although I didn't know it at the time. The lessons that I was learning the hard way would be immediately available and applicable to this essential part of my life—storing God's Word in my heart.

Under my new Captain, the ship turned around, and by the end of that dreaded semester I had moved up to the top five of the class! It seemed incredible.

Time moved along and medical school was behind me. I had completed my two-year internship and was now in my surgical residency (more of that later). My Christian experience was status quo. My spiritual ambitions had not kept pace with my educational and professional ones. *After all,* I rationalized when infrequently I would feel a prick of the Spirit, *I'm too busy to do much about Christian interests, about the things of God.*

But, one day right in the midst of such reasoning, God had a message for me, a verse that spoke to the depths in me; it was this:

> And I sought for a man among them, that should make up the hedge, and stand in the gap before me . . . but I found none.
>
> Ezekiel 22:30

This Bible verse was to have a profound, lifelong impact on me. I never got away from it.

It was a surprising new thought that God looks for *individuals.* I had always thought He dealt with people by the thousands. I found myself wondering how many there were in California of whom God could say "This is the man I'm looking for." Then I wondered about myself. It was obvious I was not such a man. Yet, in the quiet of my room I uttered this prayer, "Lord, in a small way, trusting You for the strength, *I* would like to be this kind of man."

I have since learned that there is a spiritual rule that God always takes us at our highest level of commitment. This prayer that I had breathed before God was miles above anything I had ever promised Him before. I wondered where to begin.

Would I have made my commitment, I wonder, if I could have known what God would require of me. For some, God has one way; for another, He has a different course. For me, He unquestionably showed me, it was first a matter of prayer, not one minute or five minutes a day but *one hour* early in the morning. This meant getting up at 5:30 each morning! Well, I tried it for two weeks. I didn't die. I didn't get sick. I didn't fall asleep on the job. What a tremendous blessing God had given me. It was to become a rule of life for me, never easy, but unbelievably wonderful and rewarding.

It was about nine months later that Uncle Sam welcomed me into the service—The United States Navy. Seventeen days later I was transferred to the fleet marines at Camp Pendleton (the marines obtain their doctors from the navy). After a short basic training period, we were on our way overseas, headed for the Pacific Theater.

Aboard ship was my next schoolroom where God would teach me some lessons. Twenty-seven hundred of us were packed on a ship meant for about three hundred people.

I was seated under a stairway on deck with Karl, a surgeon from the Mayo Clinic. Suddenly he turned to me with a strange request. "Tell me about the Bible," he said.

"How much of the Bible do you want to know?" I asked.

"All of it," he answered as though making an ordinary request.

Our ship was blacked out; there was no place where we could use a light at night, and in the daytime there was no time. Night it would have to be—and from *memory*. It soon became apparent that I didn't know much of the Bible. In fact you could put all I knew about it into a thimble and have room left over for your finger. As best I could, I took Karl through the Bible.

The Spirit of God really began to convince me that I had played with the Holy Scriptures. It was as if I heard God saying to me, "Begin to learn, to memorize My Word."

"But Lord, You know I can't memorize very well," I argued. (Even as I said it, I knew it wasn't true. I had put away phenomenal amounts of material in school.) Still I was mentally saying, "Forget it, God."

"Review, *review;* that's how you must learn," God seemed to say.

In turn I muttered, "But I don't *like* to memorize." This was true.

"Learn it," God said.

I remembered that I had vowed to God that I would be *such a man*. This seemed to be my marching orders. I determined to begin learning the Bible.

I tried one verse and then another, only to discover that I couldn't remember the first one. It must have sounded like "I told you so," when I complained to God that I couldn't memorize. His response was simply "Review them some more." Now I was under way in beginning to put God's Word into my heart.

There were two major things in my life that needed to be dealt with, a very bad temper, and a tendency to step on people who got in my way. The Lord simply said about these, "If you want to be the man I am looking for, get rid of these sins."

Tempers are mighty tough to control. Mine did not disappear in a blinding flash of dedication or renunciation. Though I found myself failing time and again, I was on the right road to victory over this sin as it disappeared little by little. The other trait was not such a problem to deal with, although occasionally I would find myself reverting to my old ruthless form and having to bring it to God and ask His forgiveness.

The result was spiritual strength and vigor. Salting away God's Word in my heart led to new spiritual maturity; a sensitive spirit toward my own shortcomings and sins kept me from pride and arrogance and drew me near to the Lord. He was then able to trust me as He moved me through the Pacific in a miraculous way. Things were not happening in my life by chance or good luck. God was in action.

Still, I had no idea of what God had in store for me. Meanwhile, the City of Hope was emerging as a major medical research center.

5 Split Second Timing

How much does the timing affect a situation in our lives? Looking back on those service years I can trace some incidents of split second timing, which preciseness can only be explained in terms of God's specific intervention.

One morning we had a critically wounded lieutenant brought to the hospital. His story was interesting and tragic. He was being driven in a jeep when ambushed and shot. His driver ran to safety and left him in a pool of blood. He half-fell and half-dragged himself under the jeep. There he lay for seven hours, before he was found and brought by ambulance to our hospital. His blood pressure was too low to measure, and his general condition was critical. We built him up as best we could with transfusion after transfusion. Finally we felt he was as ready for surgery as he would ever be. We began the surgery and had just identified the holes in his bowel and torn spleen when a visitor arrived. He was the head naval surgeon for the Pacific Theater. He asked what surgery we were doing. I told him that it was a gunshot wound of the abdomen. He identified himself as having been chief of surgery at the San Diego Naval Hospital before being assigned to the Pacific. I said, "How would you like to scrub in on this case and first assist me?" I was conscious of the danger involved. If he didn't like my surgery, it might mean that I would lose my job. It was a chance I would have to take. He answered, "I would love to scrub and participate. I haven't had a chance to do any surgery since I left the naval hospital." The surgery took three hours. He thanked me, said good-bye, and left. What had he thought? It was like waiting for your final exam grade. I learned later that he expressed his opinion of me in just one sentence: "That's the best young surgeon I've ever seen in the navy."

That one statement secured and stabilized my position as joint chief of surgery. I could accept this compliment without having it go to my head. Why? Because the navy captain was paying tribute to my pursuit of excellence. And this is something that God had given me as a major objective. "He hath done all things well" (Mark 7:37), the Bible tells us about Jesus.

Even so, I am convinced that God, in directing our steps, somehow sees to it, that we are in the right place at the right time with the right set of circumstances. It has never been my experience to have the Lord show me the long road ahead; rather, His leading in my life has been a step at a time. I'm aware, of course, that some people have a different experience. I know a man who, as a twelve-year-old, *knew* that God wanted him in medicine. So all through high school and college he set his sights in that direction and took all the right courses to further his education and expedite his training. He never wavered, and ultimately became what he set out to be at such a young age, a doctor.

While we are on this subject of leading and guidance, let me pause to make very clear that I'm not a person who just lives for the future. What I mean is this: ever since I realized that God has a plan for my life, I have looked for His hand in the circumstances of life. I have lived by the day, conscious of God's presence. There's a verse that says, "As thy days, so shall thy strength be" (Deuteronomy 33:25). I have a feeling that without doing harm to divine truth, we might say as thy days, so shall thy guidance be. I believe the Lord is leading us in the way we should go *whenever* we ask Him to. Nevertheless, there are the dramatic points when God intervenes to make things happen, things that will have a bearing on our future. It would take more than my ten fingers to count such instances. The case of the critically wounded lieutenant was not the first time my position was on the line.

While on Guadalcanal it had been decided that the other surgeon and I would alternate cases. Most of the cases were relatively minor and uneventful. However, a runner came to me one day and said, "One of the officers has an acute appendicitis. You are up for it!" I immediately went down to check the officer, secretly hoping that it wasn't time. However, the diagnosis was correct. In fact, it was a classic case. I scheduled surgery and prepared for the operation. All thirty-five doctors came to observe the boy from California operate. They crowded into the operating room and watched. I wasn't used to such a big audience. There was a near carnival atmosphere with lots of talking and kidding. I made the skin incision and slowly and deliberately entered the abdomen. The appendix was almost gangrenous. As I began to remove the appendix, I clamped the artery running to it and divided it. Horror of horrors occurred when the artery slipped out of the clamp, and within a split second, the wound was a sea of blood. I almost died on the spot. The operating room became deadly silent. Every eye was focused on the operative field. I was trying to decide what to do, when my assistant did what he wasn't supposed to do. He thrust a clamp into the pool of blood, and wonder of wonders, he clamped the artery. The emergency quickly came to an end, and the surgery was completed uneventfully.

How did I ever get so much responsibility? When I went into the service I was told that because of my young age, I would have to go in at the lowest rank that was given to a doctor. Because of my low rank I couldn't hope to do any surgery for at least a year. In the interim I would be a battalion aid station surgeon (a high-sounding name for a doctor doing first aid on the front lines).

Each place I was sent I kept inquiring if I could be placed in a unit where I could do surgery. Always, the answer was the same, "No chance." I spent seventeen days in the navy and was transferred to the marines. Because the doctors were being shot up with distressing rapidity, I was sent overseas almost immediately. In Pearl Harbor I was placed in the transient center to wait for final assignment. I began to pray that God would open some way to place me where I could use my training—even a little. The Lord brought to my mind Dr. H.J.S. who had been one of my professors at the University of California. I knew that he was in the navy and somewhere in the Pacific. I wondered if he might be in Pearl Harbor. There were three naval hospitals in Pearl Harbor at the time. I decided to call them. The two largest hospitals answered, "No, we don't have anyone here by that name." The third had a different answer. "Yes, Captain H.J.S. is the executive officer here, but he is back in Annapolis watching his son graduate from the academy. He will be back in three days." Here was a possible chink in the door.

I waited three days and called again. This time he answered the phone, and invited me up to see the hospital and to have lunch with him. As he showed me around, I was impressed with the excellence he had built into the hospital. The lunch was super and a high point of the day. The contrast with what I was used to eating as a marine was tremendous. I thanked Captain H.J.S. and was about to leave when he said, "One of our navy doctors in the Pacific is making the rank of commodore [one step up from a naval captain]. This is a first in this theatre." And he added, "I am in charge of the medical program."

Now one thing the Lord has taught me is that while He will frequently *make* opportunities for us, we have to *take some initiative* and make the most of such opportunities. In other words, God will open a door, but we must walk through it. This was one of those times.

Summoning up all the courage I could, I gulped, then suggested, "Sir, I'd be happy to present some of the research I did at the university on early ambulation [getting patients up early after surgery], if you wish." I waited hopefully for his answer. It was direct—and discouraging.

"Oh, I couldn't use you; your rank is too low."

Not quite daunted, I pursued it with, "If you should change your mind, sir, let me know."

Three days later I got a call from the captain. He greeted me, "I decided to take a chance and use you. Can you limit your presentation to twenty minutes?" I assured him I could. As the phone call ended, I leaped for joy. What an opportunity it was. Then the sobering thought came to me, who am I, little me, to stand before the high and the mighty. The thought made me want to run and hide.

The appointed time arrived. Suddenly I realized I had nothing to wear except my brown enlisted man's pants and shirt (both unpressed!). I did have a tie but no jacket. It didn't help much when I saw what awaited me at the hospital, two hundred high-ranking navy medical officers—all in their dress blues. As the only one not dressed for the occasion, I sat in the back of the room hoping to be inconspicuous.

Two others were before me. There was a case presentation by a lieutenant commander, a discussion by a navy captain, followed by the world's leading gastric surgeon from the Mayo Clinic. He spoke for ten minutes. Then I was introduced. I walked to the podium, flushed and nervous with my heart racing and a strange uneasiness. As I walked I could hear a ripple all over the audience: Where did they dig him up? Who is this? and What does he have on? I opened my mouth to begin, and discovered I had developed a tremor in my voice.

After a few words my voice returned to normal. Fortunately I had good material to present. Of that I was confident, even though I was at a disadvantage in having to give it purely from memory without benefit of slides or a manuscript. I'm still convinced that in my extremity, God made certain that it went well. My talk had a favorable reception as far as I could judge. Where, precisely, did God's split second timing fit into this account?

Among those who came to the presentation was the navy captain who had charge of placing all the navy doctors attached to the marines. It was the only time that he was in this hospital, but he was there this time. He introduced himself to me, and asked me to give him my full name and identification number. He wrote it down and he put it into his wallet. Ninety-nine times out of a hundred nothing ever comes of such a contact. However, four days later I received orders to go to a unit, where I would be the *surgeon*. I breathed a little prayer, "Thank You, Lord."

6 The Woman Thou Gavest Me

I have a young pastor friend who has one special sermon titled "The Call to Be Single." That sermon was not for me, as much as I regard this preacher. I never had any such call. Instinctively I knew what later I learned the Bible says, "It is not good that the man should be alone" (Genesis 2:18). I knew and felt that I would not be complete until I had a wife, the *helpmeet* heaven saw man needs for completion. In part this might have been because I observed my parents' happiness in each other.

While growing up, I would spend idle moments dreaming of the pretty girl who would one day grace my life. Certain criteria were fixed in my mind. Number one was that the girl be pretty, or more accurately, *beautiful.*

A couple of dates with good-looking girls, however, caused me to consider another top priority; none of these girls had much personality. So, to *beautiful* I added *personable,* for my dream girl. A third requirement, I decided on as I pondered on this ideal woman for me, was that she be a nice girl. In time it dawned on me that what I really had in mind was a Christian girl. But—again I had the same old hang-up. The Christian girls I had been around were just like the fellows in that they were lackluster persons; they didn't stand out as special in any way that appealed to me. Certainly none of them matched the image I had in my mind. I assumed this must be true of all Christians.

During the summer following my first year of medical school, I had a job on a road construction project. Toward the end of the summer, I had a few uncommitted days so I decided to go for some relaxation to Catalina, a resort island twenty miles off the coast of southern California. My grandmother went along too. She was fun to be with and had few wants.

The big white ship was packed with vacationers, and among them, I soon noted, were a number of attractive girls. One of them especially caught my eye. She was standing by the rail with another girl and a man and woman (later I learned they were her sister and her parents). Although I met a number of others, I didn't meet this girl aboard the ship.

Before dinner I was strolling on the island when one of the girls from the ship came toward me down the hill. "Hello, Mary," I said, thinking she was one of the girls I had met.

"My name isn't Mary," she replied.

"You told me it was," I defended myself; and she snapped back, "Oh, no I didn't. I've never even spoken to you before!"

I realized then that she was the blonde girl I had noticed but had not met.

About this time her mother appeared on the scene. There I was with my face tanned like any construction gang worker and wearing a leather jacket.

"Get rid of him," the girl's mother almost hissed, while edging up to her daughter so I wouldn't hear. But I did.

During the next thirty-six hours I saw Dorothy (that is her name) several times. We sat on the beach and on the seawall talking about anything and everything. She was friendly and sparkled as we talked. Little did I know when I boarded the ship for Los Angeles that she breathed a deep sigh of relief. Her boy friend was arriving momentarily.

Back home from my short vacation, my mother asked me if I'd met any interesting girls at Catalina. With no hesitation I answered her. "Yes," I said, "I met one I might marry some day."

It was certain that Dorothy had no such thoughts. Four months later when I was home from medical school, I decided to find Dorothy with little to go on. My two clues were her family name, DeMott, and where she lived, Culver City. Fortunately there were only two DeMotts in the phone book. I tried the wrong one first, but on my second try I contacted Dorothy and arranged a date to go roller skating. I should have thought twice about that! While

I hadn't been on roller skates for years, Dorothy had all but lived on them!

We put on our skates and took off on the rink. Then it happened! We came to the first turn; I didn't make it. My feet skidded out from under me, and down I crashed. The skaters behind me fell over me and a pileup resulted. When I finally pulled myself up with my slacks and shirt a mess, I discovered my new girl friend laughing herself silly at me. My mind flashed for a second to the time when as a toddler I had fallen in a clumsy heap. I learned that day that I didn't like to be laughed at.

Our skating date wasn't an outstanding success. I was too slow. (Apparently this didn't apply only to my roller skating. I heard later that one of Dorothy's best friends had said to another, "I don't know about that Ralph Byron. I wonder if he can handle a girl like Dorothy!") Even the infrequent times with her impressed me that I liked her more and more each time.

In South America I met a young lady, beautiful and talented with personality plus. She had it all—but she was not a Christian. I began to analyze and compare what it would be like to be married to Dorothy, a Christian, or to this non-Christian. It became apparent to me that the latter would be a disaster for me, for both of us. There would be much of her world that I could not be a part of, and she would have problems with my interests.

That fall term in San Francisco I was corresponding with both girls. That is, until November when mail from both stopped. *Horrors,* I thought when I could no longer feel it was just that the mails were slow. *Could it be that I put the letters in the wrong envelopes!* I was to learn later that I had not switched the letters, but that things had happened at the other end. Dorothy had attended a young people's conference, and had fallen in love with a young minister, fresh out of seminary; my other girl (now in the east) had gone to the Army-Navy game with a midshipman and had fallen for him.

Christmas vacation came and I dealt directly with Dorothy and she filled me in with what had happened. I asked her just one question, "Do you love this fellow?" When her reply was yes, I told her I was sure she would make an outstanding wife for a minister, and I bade her good bye. It was a sad time. But I was learning something. I now knew the kind of girl I really wanted, one like Dorothy. I found, however, that *Dorothys* were a rare breed—and the other girls I met—well, I liked them less and less. But I didn't know what the next turn in the road would bring.

That spring "when a young man's fancy lightly turns to thoughts of love," I was home from school when a longtime friend, Jack, suggested, "How about going to church with me and seeing Dorothy DeMott?"

"Dorothy! But she's engaged. Don't you know that?" I objected.

"She *was* engaged," Jack corrected me, "but it's broken off."

I hesitated. I had been hurt before. I wasn't keen to go through it again. But I agreed to go to South Hollywood Presbyterian Church, and when I saw Dorothy sitting in the choir, my heart leapt. I couldn't believe how much I liked her.

We picked up right where we had left off six months before, with this difference: this time I knew Dorothy was the girl for me. The timing was right. The Lord had taught me a little about how to treat a girl, how to be nice to her, and how to treat a girl like a queen.

Going to all her church and youth activities with Dorothy was a revelation to me. For the first time in my life I saw vital Christianity in action. Her pastor, Reverend Bob Munger, was a ball of fire who really was used by God to ignite the church people. What an eye-opener this was to me! Here was an exciting, challenging life in Christ. What I observed and, more, what I felt and experienced there, launched me into a lifelong, tremendously satisfying walk with the Lord. It was here, too, I came to know a brilliant man, a superb teacher who had only recently come to know Jesus Christ as his personal Savior. Rabbi Stein, who had been a seminary Hebrew teacher, came to Christ while reading the New Testament so he could argue against it with Christians. He held a class in Dorothy's home, and passed on some of his great insight into the Scriptures to me.

One more traumatic episode marred the otherwise smooth course of our courtship. I was in my final semester of medical school. We were separated by four hundred miles, and suddenly, again the letters stopped. *Why?* I agonized. But it was not another man this time. No, Dorothy was in the throes of having to make a major decision. Gifted with a lovely singing voice and well trained, she was being offered the world, the promise of lead roles in the New York Metropolitan Opera within two and one-half years. But—and it was a giant *but*—*You must remain single* was the stipulation.

Would she pursue a career? Would she decide that for her, happiness spelled a husband and a home? What was God's will for her? It took her a month to prayerfully make up her mind. Her decision was not to trade what she thought would bring her happiness for a career. She would get married.

It's hard to find words to describe how wonderfully God had prepared a wife for me. In so many ways, she is everything I am not. She's outgoing and very friendly; I am by nature somewhat of an introvert, shy around people. Dorothy brought me out of my shell, helped me to be comfortable around people (a necessity if others are to be comfortable with me).

Always at ease with folks, Dorothy has great talents in interpersonal relationships, and she has, through the years, imparted some of this to me. What kind of a doctor would I have been, I sometimes ponder, if God had not blessed me with just the right wife.

The Lord needs surgeons who are dedicated to their chosen profession. He can use a surgeon for whom the pursuit of excellence is a lifetime Holy Grail. But I'm reminded that without the compassion to go along with the skill, we can become about as unfeeling as the sophisticated equipment around us. I've heard it said that the word *compassion* is the nearest word to *Jesus* in all the language. I buy that. But it took my wife—bless her—to teach me the importance of the humanity, the *compassion* factor. She was the one who helped me to activate the Bible verses I had memorized.

Another of Dorothy's great assets is her ability in decision making. There were times when very important decisions had to be made. Major steps became *our* steps, not just my steps. When I was faced with the option of taking my surgical residency in Los Angeles or San Francisco, it was Dorothy who wisely asked, "Where will you get the better training?" "Probably in San Francisco," I answered, and she said, "Well, that settles it."

"But," I argued for her sake more than for my own, "it would mean leaving our nice new little apartment and our families and our friends. Are you sure you want to do that?"

"I've thought about all that," she insisted. "But we must go where it will be best for you."

Dorothy has been and is a super help to me spiritually. She has a practical, God-given wisdom in spiritual matters. When we were dating, we always prayed together before we parted; we grew spiritually together. And God made us one in this all-important area of our lives through our marriage. I look back and it seems unbelievable that God would do all this for me, prepare the right girl for me—the one who is above and beyond anything I could ever have hoped for. Every man should be so blessed!

Dorothy and I had been free to go where we wanted and do as much or as little as we wished. We were limited only by time and that critical ingredient, money. This all changed with dramatic suddenness in the form of a blonde, bouncy little girl—Joanne! It was immediately apparent that we would have to reprogram our lives. Nothing was simple anymore. There were diapers, play-pens, formula, and a million little things to think about every time we went anyplace.

I had done an unofficial study of ministers' and missionaries' children to decide in my own mind what went wrong in a significant number of such families. (It was not difficult to get data apart from my own observations, since the role of physician tends to make one the repository of other people's problems and frustrations.)

One conclusion I came to is that somehow, in the busy life of the minister and missionary their children are left out. In some, this breeds resentment that the parents love the Lord but don't love the child. In time it can lead to spiritual dropouts and to the parents' lamenting, "We did everything we could; what went wrong?"

Actually *what went wrong* was that the parents were often *too* busy doing good things for the Lord. Dorothy and I decided we wouldn't let this happen. We would simply take Joanne everywhere. If people wanted us, they would have to accept our baby also.

It was at this time that I had become interested in early ambulation of patients in the postoperative period. What was more natural than to apply my know-how in teaching Joanne to walk early? Between Dorothy's natural ability with babies and my know-how, Joanne walked alone, four days before she was eight months old. I immediately concluded she must be a genius! She was not; she was bright but of normal intelligence and had reacted favorably to being pushed in this one area of development.

Joanne was fifteen months old when I was welcomed into the United States Marine Corps. I wondered if she would remember me; if, indeed, I would ever see her again, and how long it would be before I was reunited with her and her wonderful mother, God's great gift to me.

7 How Did I Ever Get into This?

Active duty overseas isn't always blood, sweat, and tears. Our first few weeks on Okinawa were almost as leisurely as a vacation. Oh, the chow was awful, the weather foul, and living conditions didn't approximate a pleasure cruise. But, to compensate, casualties were light and surgery was unhurried rather than emergency. I began to wonder, *Is this war?*

Then it happened! How can I describe the next thirty days? With a steady flow of wounded, I operated around the clock. As the days dragged on, I became unbelievably tired. Between cases I was almost asleep on my feet, but somehow as I began the operation, I was able to mobilize sufficient alertness to function as a surgeon.

My assistants and corpsmen were equally beat. They were little more than boys, barely eighteen and just out of high school. Their *training* was a few weeks at the San Diego Naval Hospital; their surgical experience was a couple of hemorrhoidectomies and a few minor surgeries. They were destined to grow up in a hurry. I was trying to cram four years of medical school, two years of internship, and three years of surgical training into boys who had not even entered college—and I was attempting to do it in one month. "The difficult we do immediately; the impossible takes a little longer." I recalled the air force slogan.

I was surprised at how much of my professors' knowledge I had soaked up; how maybe the endless months of training had been worthwhile after all. I found myself smiling as I shared not only surgical procedures, but attitudes, ways to give patients the best, and how to put tender loving care into action. It was hard to know how much they understood, how much they grasped, or how much they would remember.

In the life and death urgency of the situation I would make my way from surgery—gown, gloves, and all—straight to the chapel. There I would share with the men the matchless Gospel, that Jesus is God who has moved into history and borne our sins and died that we might have everlasting life. Faith in Christ as Savior and Lord is the only answer. There are no alternatives.

Scores of the wounded wouldn't make it. There would be no welcome home parades and bands for them. This is a foregone conclusion of war. As I worked over them I couldn't help but wonder if they had mothers who had taught them about God and Jesus Christ. Had some, I mused, once trusted the Lord, but had the pull of the world drawn them, like the Prodigal Son, into the far country?

None of us, the still unscathed, could be certain we would see another sunrise. There was a desperation; no time to linger in the valley of indecision. Nothing was more important than sounding out a clear, easy-to-understand Christian message.

The response was gratifying. I found that the wounded were impressed that I felt this was really important or I wouldn't have been there. The reward was the joy of seeing young men come to Christ. Was it worth the extra effort? Yes, infinitely so!

The war continued. With the hectic regime my weight began to drop. I lost fifteen pounds. I caught myself wondering why I ever decided to go into surgery. How did I ever get myself into such a position?

How did I? I couldn't know it, but God was, step-by-step, moving me in the direction of His will for my life. And this was a part of it.

It was while I was in a two-year rotating internship that I began to gradually have the conviction that God wanted me in surgery. But just the process of applying to the Los Angeles General Hospital was almost enough to discourage me completely. I lined up the required letters of recommendation—took the oral exam, which was something between an inquisition and the last defense before the gallows—and, wonder of wonders, I got the residency. It did not solve the riddle of my future, however.

Knowing the strong competition for surgical residencies, I had applied simultaneously to Los Angeles County and to my medical alma mater, the University of California in San Francisco. Of course the latter was foolish. I knew it, for when I had asked the professor of surgery there, "If I intern in Los Angeles, could I return here for my surgical residency?" his answer was a curt "no." If you go down there, I'm through with you." Nevertheless, after praying about it, I decided to write. I lumped my assets for the position into three cryptic sentences:

> My health is good.
> Finances are not a problem.
> You know my record.

There was no response for nearly six months then—a comedy of errors! An opportunity for an interview came, but I was so engrossed in my work at Los Angeles General County Hospital that I forgot until it was almost too late to arrange it. I was already late in starting out to keep the appointment when a freak, torrential rain snarled traffic. When I finally arrived, Dr. N. greeted me with, "Where in blazes have you been, Byron? You'll have to come back tomorrow." "Can't," I replied. "I'm on call."

"I remember you well as a student, but my associate, Dr. H.B., was away the year you were a senior and doesn't remember you. Will you phone him in the morning?" I agreed and made, what I thought to be, the unimportant call. I was sure that any chance of a residency in San Francisco had evaporated.

A week went by; then came a telegram. I had been appointed assistant resident in surgery, University of California Medical School in San Francisco. My former professor, who said "You can never come back," would be directing my steps in surgery.

No residencies in surgery—now I had two! Which to accept? The decision was a tough one. The Los Angeles residency was three and one-half sure years. The San Francisco program was a year to year appointment and the professor said, "I will frankly admit that if a better man comes along, I will drop you and appoint him." Also, going to San Francisco meant uprooting my new wife from our cute little apartment and taking her away from the town near her parents to a strange new environment. After praying about it, I asked my wife, "What do you think?" She said, "If you think it will be better for you in San Francisco, I'm ready to go." Although I wasn't sure why, I felt we should go. We moved our handful of belongings, found an apartment, and I plunged into the grueling cutthroat competition of the residency that was to be a major part of my preparation for my lifework.

I've pondered many times what course my life would have taken, how much I would have missed, if my wife were not the great person she is. What if she, understandably enough, had balked at being uprooted so early in our marriage; what if she had discouraged the move to San Francisco? She didn't. But all that was before Uncle Sam invited me into his service.

There would be many times that I would wonder why I ever got into surgery. Was it for the spiritual opportunities this service would afford? Was this where God needed a man to *stand in the gap?* That day when with little to offer, I had made my commitment to be *such a man* with God's help, He was looking ahead to World War II. Had He already prepared a place where I could combine the physical and the spiritual? For, gratifying as it is to have a part in easing a man's pain and prolonging his life, ultimately "it is appointed unto men once to die" (this is one appointment we must all keep), "but after this the judgment" (Hebrews 9:27).

We were rarely aware of how the battle was going, confined as we were to our makeshift hospitals. But we weren't alone in our ignorance. As the great war correspondent Ernie Pyle used to comment, "It is impossible for a soldier in the front lines to know more about the battle than two hundred yards on either side of him." So we listened to the discouraging reports as we pumped the men brought in from the lines. Always the answers to my question, "How is the battle going?" added up to, "We're being beaten bad."

I could hardly believe it when the announcement came: "The island is secured; the battle is over." Naturally, my sigh of relief was mixed with some curiosity and—yes—excitement. What lay ahead? I would soon find out. The United States Marine Corps had my life mapped for the immediate future. More importantly, I was about to receive God's ongoing orders.

8 Is *That* in the Bible?

Although my life was full of activity, to my mind frequently came my promise made to God, that I was willing to be His man *standing in the gap*. I was about to have my opportunity.

Our training was complete, our equipping procedure ended and we were at full staff. Like many cattle we were herded aboard a former round-the-world-cruise luxury liner, now a troop carrier. She was jammed to the gunnels. Because of the danger of submarines or air attacks we, the thirty-five doctors, supporting troops, and equipment, had been split into three groups and put on three different ships. This way one successful torpedo would not get us all—a nice thought!

After a number of days in which we practiced convoying, only to find ourselves anchored back in the harbor the next morning, we were awakened by the roll of the ship. This time it was for real. We were under way.

About half-past three in the afternoon there was an announcement: The chaplain invites all troops to a sing on the fantail of the ship.

I attended. We sang some good old hymns—and were dismissed. Some thirty fellows had been present. At the conclusion I approached the two chaplains—a ship's chaplain was aboard as well as our troop chaplain—and I made a suggestion. "With just a few changes this sing could become an evangelistic meeting; and I would be glad to help in any way I could." A moment of silence, then the ship chaplain spoke up. "Would you be willing to meet with me in my office at eight this evening?"

Would I? My hopes soared as I replied, "Sure, I'll be there."

Promptly at eight, I presented myself. I was greeted by this chaplain with the direct question, "What are you trying to do, Byron: steal my job?"

Nonplussed I responded, "No, Chaplain. I have no such idea." Regaining my thoughts I added, "I am very conscious that many of these men may be killed in the near future; I'm anxious that they hear the Gospel before they die."

He turned on me saying "You don't mean to tell me you, a medical doctor, believe all that stuff, that the Bible is the Word of God?" My answer, "I most certainly do," was the signal for a word volley.

"You believe all of it?'

"All of it."

"Job?"

"Yes, Job."

"Jeremiah?"

"Yes, Jeremiah."

"Genesis?"

"Yes, Genesis."

The chaplain was beginning to raise his voice. He next switched to a philosophical denial of various books of the Bible. When he came to Genesis, his attack was, "What about the two different accounts of creation in the first and second chapters of Genesis?"

"These are not different accounts," I batted back. "They simply supplement one another in the same way that the four Gospel accounts team up to give us a complete picture of Jesus and His ministry." I then suggested we get down on our knees and pray about the whole thing.

"Pray! Oh, I don't believe in that kind of prayer," he countered.

I tried another tack. "Which parts of the Bible *do* you believe in as the Word of God?"

"Matthew, Mark, Luke, and parts of Peter," he told me.

"All right. I will confine my quoting to that portion of the Bible," I said. Then I probed, "What do you think of the words of Jesus, 'Think not that I am come to destroy the law, or the prophets: I am not come to destroy, but to fulfil. For verily I say unto you, Till heaven and earth pass, one jot or one tittle shall in no wise pass from the law, till all be fulfilled' " (Matthew 5:17, 18).

"Is *that* in the Bible?" he asked.

"Oh, yes," I answered. My mind was going a mile a minute. If ever there was a *hole in the hedge,* a *gospel gap* that needed to be filled, surely this was it—and the men aboard ship would be the victims of it. *There must be something I could do,* I thought. I had an idea!

"Chaplain," I said. "Your biggest meeting with the men is your Sunday chapel service. That's where you get up and you give your greatest message. I'd like to suggest that when you finish, you give an invitation; *some* kind of invitation. Invite the men to write their mothers on Sunday, if you like. Then let me have equal time. I'll give a simple Gospel message then I, too, will give an invitation. I'll invite the fellows to accept the Savior. We will see which invitation God blesses."

"Oh, you'll obviously win, Byron; you have something definite to say." (This chaplain had been a seminary professor, and a pastor of a church for some years.)

Before we parted I said I felt the time was not quite right for the meetings, but that when I did feel it was the time, I would ask his permission.

"As long as I'm chaplain of this ship," he answered, "I'll *never* permit you to have such meetings. I've had experience with over-zealous religionists and how you try to wreck my ministry."

Quite calmly I repeated, "Chappy, when I feel it's time I will come and ask your permission to put on the meetings. If you say no, I'll go ahead with them anyway."

Meanwhile, I had made an acquaintance with two Christian fellows. We found a place below decks where we could meet; so at nine o'clock each night on a corrugated iron floor, we would kneel down and pray together. The two grew to ten, then twenty-five, and I longed that it might be an evangelistic meeting so that some would find Christ as Savior. To my amazement, unsaved men came and some accepted Christ and were born again. When I saw how God was directing in our nightly prayer meeting, I began to give an invitation and time after time there were decisions.

About this time we learned that our fourteen-hundred-ship convoy was headed for Okinawa. I sensed this was God's time for me to make a move in the direction of evangelistic meetings.

It was a Sunday morning at nine o'clock. I visited the ship chaplain in his cabin. "Chappy," I began, "I told you that when I felt the time was right for evangelistic meetings, I would come and ask your permission. I think the time is now." Silence.

"Will you give me a half hour to make up my mind?"

A half hour later we were in the regular chapel service. The chaplain was pale and perspiring; there was a tremor in his voice as he stated,

"Men! A month ago I was sure I would never make this announcement. Now I'm informing you that there will be evangelistic services on the fantail of the ship. Dr. Byron will be in charge, and I not only give him permission, but will furnish my public address system and cooperate in every way possible."

What an answer to prayer! I was ready to throw my arms around the chaplain and hug him.

There was still one more major hurdle, however. I had to obtain permission from the captain of our ship. I made my way to the bridge, and faced this venerable officer with my request. He looked hard at me. Then slowly, thoughtfully, he shook his head and explained, "The amphibian commander has issued an order that no mass meetings be held on any ship because of the great submarine and air attack danger: if I say yes to your request, it will be the only such meeting on any of the fourteen hundred ships."

I held my breath.

A long moment, then—"I say *YES.*"

Each afternoon the meetings were put on, and although rain is so common in that part of the tropics, the Lord gave us fine weather. About one hundred troops came to the first meeting, and as the message began to pass by word of mouth through the ship, each day saw fellows deciding for Christ. Many of them were never to see home again, but they were ready to meet the Lord.

One night in our prayer meeting I was especially aware that nobody was praying, "Don't let me get hit, Lord"; rather their prayer was, "Help me during the invasion and the battle ahead to show Jesus in my life." What a way to pray!

At three the next morning (typical marine corps timing) we

were shouted awake with the loudspeaker blaring the captain's terse message: "Get dressed and ready to go ashore!" Then we were served a meal that made us feel as though the galley crew thought it would be our last on earth—steak, lamb chops, and apple pie a la mode.

We were ordered to board the landing craft as our names were called. I thought I must be hearing things when the crisp *Byron* was the first name called. *Surely it must be a mistake,* I thought. *No one in his right mind would send a doctor in first.* But no, the marines send the doctors ashore first so that they can be ready for the casualties. What a great idea!

One thing about that before-dawn disembarkment is a treasured memory. As the boat with me in it was lowered over the side of the troop carrier, the ship's chaplain leaned over the rail and called to me, "I want you to know, Dr. Byron, that you have helped me more than any person since I became a Christian. I am going back to America *with a message.*"

This amazed me at the time because all I had done was be a friend to him and share the Word of God with him.

9 The Fateful August 2

Our next assignment was Guam, and we were to travel by air. Since that day I have spent many hours waiting for a plane, but never did the waiting have the significance for me that it did that day. I was able to find a quiet spot where I reflected and read my Bible. I had seen the horrors of war; had been a part of suffering and death. And I had learned valuable lessons. What, I speculated, did God have for me to learn from my next experience?

Always, at such times of reflection, I wondered when God was going to give me specific direction, His marching orders for me to *stand in the gap*. That day I was musing, will it be China, India, Africa, or the islands of the Pacific (I had seen plenty of need there). *Where,* Lord? Where do You want to use me?

That I had God's ear that day could never be disputed. He spoke to me as directly, through His Word, as He had spoken to the prophet Ezekiel in his day:

> For thou art not sent to a people of a strange speech and of an hard language, but to the house of Israel.
>
> Ezekiel 3:5

Here was my answer. I wrote alongside the verse, August 2, 1945. It was the second time that God had given me a verse that strongly influences me to this day.

In my professional life I tend to be always looking for a better way to do things (maybe I'm a tinkerer at heart). One such example of discontent with my work led to my first piece of published research in my service days. While I was in Guam, it bothered me that some of my surgical knots did not stay tied. Now a rest period gave me opportunity to think about this, and I was determined to find out the reason. It definitely was a homemade experiment. From a two-by-four-inch board, a spring, a nail, and an improvised crank, I constructed a thread tester and experimented with it innumerable times. I recorded my findings and ultimately resolved the problem. And no one was more surprised than I when this piece of research appeared in the *Naval Medical Bulletin*. It came to be known as "The Classic on Knots."

Where there is a doctor there usually is a potential patient. A number of the men had tattoos which after a change of mind, they wanted removed. I volunteered my services and though I didn't hit on the best method, I was able to remove them successfully by multiple excisions. I learned in a hurry that there is a limit to how much skin will stretch even when the procedure is carried out over a series of weeks. These other activities had their place, but I was anxious to get the Gospel to our marines.

On Guadalcanal some fellow Christians and I had hit on a plan that worked. Fewer than 15 percent of the men there attended chapel services, Catholic and Protestant. Obviously, the chapel was not the place to reach them. What was there to do? It came to me that if the Gospels teach anything, they teach that Jesus went *where the people were*. Night after night *where the marines were*—about 100 percent of them—was the picture show. So we devised our strategy: we obtained permission from the commanding officer and the chaplain, and proceeded. Twenty minutes before and twenty minutes into show time we sang a hymn such as "The Old Rugged Cross" (which so many seemed to appreciate singing), recited a verse of Scripture from memory, then delivered a hard-hitting Gospel message for about thirty-eight minutes, and had an invitation at the end. I saw as many as two hundred men make a decision for Christ in a single evening! Originally the meetings were billed as *Old Fashioned Revival Meetngs,* till the Lord showed me a better line, *Spiritual Combat Conditioning Meetings*. I should add that I'm no hero; it took all the courage I could muster to stand before two thousand rough, tough marines who had come to see a movie—and present the Gospel to them!

I can see that through such experiences the Lord was helping me to find creative ways to witness for Him in *impossible* situations. There would be plenty such situations, I have learned. And God has moved in with one of His miracles and honored my efforts when I've taken some step. How truly it has been said that God can only direct a *moving* object.

Knowing our plan worked, while we were in Guam we asked permission to conduct the same kind of meeting at a large neighboring outfit. The weather threatened to torpedo our efforts. Tropical rain is of two kinds, the short daily downpour in the afternoon and the rain storm that lasts for days. An hour before our scheduled meeting, a torrential rain started. What were we to do? Why should we even bother since the best movie wouldn't hold an audience in this storm? was the consensus of our team. While my head agreed with them, I couldn't settle for not going. I shared with them my feelings that the meeting was vital; that the men desperately needed a chance to hear the Gospel. Then I suggested, "Let's pray that God will take care of the rain." We prayed then climbed into an open truck; the rain continued unabated. Then, as we arrived at the place, a band of blue appeared overhead. Right where we were it had stopped raining, but we could see that it was still pouring down on either side of us. The men came, and God met with us. Many decisions were made for Christ that night. Then, the meeting over, the rainstorm pelted down, washing out the show that was to follow, and it continued for three days. God had sent His band of blue, not only that some might hear and be saved, but I believe that He did it to encourage us to *believe* in the God of the miraculous.

News of the first atomic bomb came over the Armed Forces Radio. We couldn't believe there could be such a bomb. Was it just propaganda? Then came the descriptions of the atomic device in New Mexico, the melting of the tower, and the fusing of the ground.

Immediately, upon hearing of the awesome fact, the horrifying implications of such a bomb, my mind swept to what the Bible says in 2 Peter 3:10:

> But the day of the Lord will come as a thief in the night; in the which the heavens shall pass away with a great noise, and the elements shall melt with fervent heat . . . .

It was the next verse that made me dash over to the chaplain and point out to him that he should preach on this *atomic bomb* topic the next Sunday. For the next verse goes on to warn, "Seeing then that all these things shall be dissolved, what manner of persons ought you to be . . ." (2 Peter 3:11).

"I don't understand about all that," the chaplain countered.

"I'm not sure I do either," I admitted, "but I'll brief you as much as I can." The timely sermon was well received. Afterwards one of the doctors came to me and said, "It's obvious who wrote that sermon."

Aware that our world had entered a new era, I speculated as to the changes that would be made, if medicine would be affected, and what God had in store for me next.

My strong faith in God was well mixed with a sense of the practical; I was always on the lookout for ways to do things better. I learned in the process that a man's own ingenuity can sometimes get him into difficulties. Here is a classic example.

We doctors had been encouraged to carry our own instruments. By nature I was a collector and I had assembled a fine array of instruments, some from the marines, some from the army, some from the navy, and some sent from home. It was a super collection. Then the question arose as to where I should put them and how I would carry them around. Well, a corpsman solved that problem for me. He made a wooden box, which was reinforced and very heavy. Loaded with instruments it was almost more than I could carry. It was my constant companion for a year and a half and created some near disasters as I would ascend and descend the dangling rope ladders on the side of a ship.

On one occasion as I climbed aboard a makeshift hospital ship, I was met by the head medical officer. He immediately wanted to know what was in the strange, gray, wooden box I was carrying. I opened it and showed him two sets of sterile instruments which were all ready for important surgery. He was impressed beyond words and falsely assumed that I was a high ranking, brilliantly trained general surgeon. (Before leaving our troop ship we had been advised that our officer's insignia worn on the collar made us prime targets for enemy snipers; so we hid the telltale markers under our collars.) Thus, the only clue as to my qualifications was my box of instruments, and although this medical officer was better trained than I, he made me chief of surgery. With such credentials, the ship's surgeon was content to let me do the surgery, give the orders, and generally run the show! I was delighted.

The first cases were straightforward and uncomplicated. They went well. I gained confidence quickly. Then, as so often happens, pride goes before a fall; the roof caved in.

A critically wounded young man was brought aboard. He was in deep shock. We worked feverishly to get him out of shock and ready for surgery. We transfused him repeatedly, but his condition failed to improve. As a desperate last resort we took him to surgery, amputated the badly torn leg, and repaired the gaping wounds. When we finished the surgery, the boy was dead. I was devastated. Throughout my training I had always been protected from such a happening.

To make matters worse, the ship's surgeon began to criticize me. It was at this moment he accidentally discovered that he outranked me. It was a crisis of the greatest magnitude. It looked like—and could have spelled—the end of my surgical career.

Again, God had His hand on my life. Before this superior could take any action against *the impostor* (me, although it was all unwitting on my part) orders arrived for me to go ashore. Wonder of wonders, he decided to drop the matter. He even bade me a friendly good-bye and wished me luck.

Once again my box and I climbed with difficulty into a small boat and headed for the beach. This time it was for real! As I approached the shore, I knew that the danger around me was growing by the minute. However, I knew that God was with me. He had given me a quiet inner confidence that there was not a bullet made that could hit me, unless He permitted it. The words of Jesus kept ringing in my innermost thoughts, "I will never leave thee, nor forsake thee" (Hebrews 13:5). "Lo, I am with you alway, even unto the end of the world" (Matthew 28:20). This was more than enough.

No one can be sure how he will react to extreme danger, heavy bombings, flak, and death on every side. As we had approached D-day we had tried to predict which of the thirty-five doctors might fall apart under the pressure. Obviously, we didn't know but no one thought he would be the one. We had predicted that one doctor, who was a frail slip of a young man with artistic hands and a quiet unimpressive carriage would go to pieces under pressure. There was a second doctor, a neurosurgeon who was brilliant, outgoing, and confident to the point of being cocky, with a great muscular physique; he would certainly stand like the Rock of Gibraltar. How wrong we were. Our frail little doctor was magnificent under the heaviest of fire. He ran the admitting room in an impeccable fashion. Our brainy neurosurgeon collapsed and had to be evacuated. Our vocal, self-confident ear, nose, and throat man was so scared he broke his toe running for his foxhole.

Our first crisis came all too soon. We were operating late at night, the patient's abdomen was open; surgery was progressing satisfactorily when a monstrous air raid came. (I think the enemy planes mistook us for something more important.)

As the bombs began to fall and the antiaircraft flak started to rain, my anesthetist, first assistant, and two corpsmen ran for their foxholes. I was left with a wounded soldier in the midst of his surgery. If I deserted him, he would either die or be disastrously affected by being left in such a state. There was only one thing to do; finish the operation. Twenty minutes later, as I was putting the last stitch in, the *all clear* sounded. My team came back, asking what happened to the patient. I took the occasion to admonish them and told them, "If we are going to die, it will be at the operating table, not running for a foxhole!" They never ran again.

10 China Adventure—and Then Home

The dropping of the atomic bombs dramatically ended the war. Mingled with our surprise and delight were the questions, how soon do I go home and how quickly can I get out of the service? It had been *so long* since I had seen my Dorothy and mail is a poor substitute at best. And what of our little Joanne, would she know me?

The Marines could have sent us home. They didn't. Rather than routing us east and toward home, for us it was west—and China. *China.* I was reminded of my prayer for direction said some months before: "Lord, where is your field of service for me; is it China?"

On board ship (jammed as usual) three of us stood huddled as we looked over the ocean toward the great land of China. We held a little prayer meeting then and there. The crux of it was, "Lord, we want to reach China for You. Help us *by whatever miracle;* You know we can't speak a word of Chinese."

Ours was a triumphal entry with little boats coming to meet us as we reached harbor and American and Chinese flags flying. The same welcome greeted us as we traveled by train to the city of Tientsin. The cheering and the waving of the crowds reminded me of the Tournament of Roses Parade in Pasadena!

My position was joint chief of surgery at the British General Hospital, a sixteen-bed facility with a surgery and X-ray setup. We had barely arrived when one of our marines cut the tendon in his hand. I had my instruments but the anesthetics had not yet been unloaded. I went from hospital to hospital in this city of more than one million people and all that was available was 8 cubic centimeters (cc's) of local anesthesia. It was essential then that I do a successful nerve block the first time and complete the surgery before the anesthetic wore off. Failure could be a minor disaster. To my relief, everything worked perfectly; the tendon was repaired—and I breathed my "thank You again, Lord."

A message came from the general asking that I see a patient in consultation with the local doctors. I went to the home of the patient, a child, saw him, and met the doctors. Both were older than I and had much more training. To make matters worse, the patient had a condition which I didn't know much about. It didn't help much when I learned that the treatment which I was somewhat familiar with had already been given. Feeling woefully inadequate inside, I nevertheless determined not to show it. I did a very deliberate examination, offered a few words of wisdom, answered several questions, and made a hasty exit. I had survived the consultation! That called for another thank-you.

But what of the spiritual opportunities? Hadn't God heard our prayer on the high seas en route to China? Weren't we to have a chance to share the Gospel?

As I walked the streets, to my mind would come the hymn "Where Cross the Crowded Ways of Life." Crowds! They spilled over from the sidewalks that could not hold them. The rickshaws jostled each other, making travel on the streets all but impossible. Hundreds—thousands—of Chinese, and they couldn't understand a word I said, nor could I understand them. How could we possibly reach them?

Then, I was walking down the street when I felt a tap on my left shoulder. It was a middle-aged Chinese woman, and she introduced herself simply as, "I'm a doctor. How would you like a place to hold meetings, a place seating twelve hundred—and heated." (This last was almost unbelievable; so few places were heated.)

In amazement I could only stammer, "I accept. Where is it?"

The woman explained, "It is the Wesley Methodist Church auditorium," then she bade me good-bye. I never saw her again. It was no problem for me to believe then that God had done the miraculous; He *had* heard our shipboard prayer.

The church was indeed available to us weekly. We were now on the right track. What were we to call our meetings? About that time a clipping in my mail told of the success of the Chicago Youth For Christ. So why not call our services Tientsin Youth For Christ?

We launched quite an advertising program in that Chinese city, newspapers, radio, and large placards. They carried the name, location, and time, along with "Lieutenant Ralph L. Byron, Jr., speaker." (I couldn't know the trouble this would get me into!) We placed five hundred signs in store windows, public bulletin boards, and even on the back of rickshaws. It gave us a particular kick to see a Buddhist priest riding along in a rickshaw advertising our Christian meetings!

The China Inland Mission with whom we consulted assured us that everyone was interested in learning English, and they would come just to practice their English. With this in mind we announced that the meeting would be in English, and some six hundred Chinese attended the first one. It was soon evident that they didn't understand what I was saying, and at the invitation the sole response was from a marine who committed his life to Christ. It was particularly distressing to see only blank looks on the faces of the Chinese. Our second try, a week later, attracted just one hundred. *What a fizzle,* I thought sadly.

My two marine buddies who helped most in organizing the meetings were sent home; their overseas duty was completed. I was left alone with my evangelistic endeavor falling around my ears. But that was not my most immediate problem!

The commanding officer sent for me. I went to his office immediately. His message was terse: "You, Lieutenant Byron, are being brought up for court-martial."

"Who, me! Why—what—," I stammered. *"Court martial!"*

"Don't you realize what you have done: you, an American officer, have your name splashed on placards all over this city as speaker, organizer, and director of some kind of religious meetings?" It was all too obvious that my commanding officer was reacting violently to what (I learned later) a navy captain had seen and had reported to him.

I was about-facing to leave when this officer said, "You have *one* chance to escape court-martial. *Stop* these meetings—and the charges will be dropped."

I went to my room, and reviewed the situation with the Lord

while on my knees. If I am court-martialed, all of the non-Christian doctors and friends to whom I had witnessed would say, "There you are, that fool religion ruined you; we knew that your fanaticism would get you into trouble." I spent most of the night praying and asking God for His perfect will on the matter.

Suddenly while I was on my knees, the Lord brought to my remembrance what Abraham had done when God asked him to offer Isaac, his son, his most precious earthly possession, as a sacrifice. It struck me that my most precious possession in Tientsin was my job as chief of surgery. It was more important than money or any material thing I had. It was a miracle that I had it. Was I willing to give it back to God, to offer it as a sacrifice? The decision was not easy. I liked my job. It gave me prestige; it allowed me to do the kind of surgery I liked; I desperately wanted to keep it. My big decision came in the early hours of the morning. "All right, Lord, You gave it to me; You may have it back; I *will* put on another meeting. Certainly the need is here; the preliminaries have been carried out, the basic structuring of the meetings has been developed."

Hardly had I made my decision when the Lord gave me an idea. Why not speak through an interpreter?

Immediately I set out to get an interpreter. We found our man, Mr. T.C. He was Chinese, a committed Christian, had gone to Wheaton College in Illinois, and had a winsome, flashing smile. There was one problem. He spoke poor Chinese (for the local area) and did not speak English very well either. Nevertheless, we advertised (more signs!) that our meeting would be in both English and Chinese. More than nine hundred Chinese came. Of these, six made a decision to accept Jesus Christ as Savior and Lord. The following week brought twelve hundred and thirty-three decisions. We were under way. That prayer meeting aboard ship had not gone unnoticed.

God had an interesting way of taking care of my court-martial. Whatever good my name would do had already been accomplished. There was no need for me to use it anymore. They could pull down all the posters that were still up if they wished. The matter of my running the meetings was easily solved. I had twenty Chinese Christians act as a board of directors to run the meetings.

They elected me chairman. I continued to run the meetings as before but officially they were run by the committee. Oh, yes!—the navy captain, what happened to him? He got the worst eye infection that I have ever seen. He had to be evacuated to the States! With no one to press the charges—they were dropped!

Five and one-half months after arriving in China, my orders came to return home. Even with the building excitement of going home to my wife and my little daughter, there was a certain sadness associated with leaving the flourishing work for God and new found friends. The Chinese Christians were like my own family. They had a going-away party for me with a sumptuous meal. For entertainment they had the new Christians give their testimonies in Chinese and translated them into English for me. One boy said, "Three weeks ago I took Christ as my Savior, two weeks ago my brother accepted Christ, and last week my father came to the Lord." Needless to say, it was exciting entertainment.

As we left, the pulsating thought came; will God *now* reveal His plan? We boarded ship and set sail for the States. We entered Yokohama, Tokyo's harbor, but were not allowed off the boat. (The day would come when I would return.) On the high seas one of the men developed appendicitis and had to be taken to our makeshift surgery. It was quite an experience for me to be pushed away from the operating table by the roll of the ship. However, as my professor had said, "It isn't a question of whether you can or can't do it, you *have* to do it." The boy survived the surgery without incident.

One day two of the doctors came to me and said, "We have a marine with a strange rash. Will you look at him?" I went to the sick bay and found a young man with a classic case of German measles. I said to my colleagues, "You'd better let me take care of him. I'm immune to everything." After working in the contagious disease section of the county hospital for three months as an intern, I was certain I was now immune to everything.

We were somewhat concerned about possible changes in our wives and children. All sort of stories filtered through to us in the islands. My regular mail, however, relieved any negative expectations. It was soon apparent that *my* wife had not changed, but was more lovely than ever. What about my three-year-old daughter?

She had been just fifteen months old when I left. Her mother had shown her my picture with some regularity. Even so, when one of my fellow officers arrived home ahead of me he went to say hello to my wife. He rang the bell; my little Joanne opened the door, and then went running into the kitchen yelling, "My Daddy's home. My Daddy is home!" She had been looking at the *uniform* all these months, not the face in the picture.

The first few hours I was delighted to discover my daughter wanted to stay with me, do things with me, and be my constant pal. How wrong the overseas reports had been. Then it happened, the new toy wore out; Joanne would have nothing to do with me. It would be many weeks before I would really be her father. I had to earn it.

I couldn't understand then and indeed for some time, just what was going on in that little girl's head. From her point of view I came along and made her share her mother whom, up until now, she had all to herself. She obviously resented this—and I didn't help my cause one little bit when, on occasion, I had to discipline her.

And that immunity I had bragged about? That was a joke. I arrived home, and twenty-four hours later I had a blotchy rash. I had caught German measles, and promptly gave them to Joanne.

11 Meet the *Little Corporal*

At the age of ten, Dorothy DeMott said to her mother, "I'm going to marry a doctor." Yet by her own admission, she "couldn't stand doctors" (with the exception of a kindly, old family physician).

What is it like being the wife of a world-renowned surgeon, who is practically a walking Bible and whose driving aim in life is the pursuit of excellence? Here talented, attractive, vivacious Mrs. Ralph Byron shares some of what she describes as "thirty-five super years."

In the early years it wasn't quite the life I planned. Of course I had known that my husband would be on call—but midnight or later night after night! I remember complaining (petulantly, as I think of it now), "Ralph, you *want* to be away from me; you'd rather be at that hospital!"

Well, I can remember it still. Ralph sat me down and said, "You might as well get this straight, Dorothy. My work *must* come first. Now I'm not saying I love my work first, but I am involved with people's lives. That's how it's always going to be."

Just like that he told me, direct with no preamble. That's Ralph. "I *love you,*" he assured me. "I want you to feel secure in my love and have faith in me."

Undoubtedly some of my negative feelings stemmed from the fact that we had moved from everything that was dear and familiar to me; I had never lived away from Los Angeles before. But San Francisco was where Ralph's finest opportunity was, and I was only too happy to make the move. However, on a resident's shoestring pay all we could afford was a rather dismal old apartment, furnished with the few pieces of furniture we had brought with us. The windows were ten-feet high, and in an attempt to brighten my surroundings, I went bargain shopping for drapes. I found some in a store basement—for $4.95. They weren't what I would have bought if money had been no object, but I was pleased with the improvement the colorful drapes made. I was eager for Ralph to see how nice I had fixed them. When he came home he *laughed*. "They're too short," he said and laughed some more. They were short by a foot, but they were the longest we could afford. I got mad, packed my suitcase, and left. I spent a desperately lonely night in a hotel, hurting more by the hour. Ralph, meanwhile, spent the night trying all the places I might be. Somehow, he missed one hotel.

Because we truly love each other, the problem was short-lived. It sorted itself out the next day. Like many other struggling young doctors' wives, I worked in the hospital (for thirty-five dollars a month!). Ralph sought me out there and we made up.

It was an impulsive, immature thing I did, but from it I learned some worthwhile lessons. I can understand and empathize with the frustrations of the student's wife who came to me with her troubles. She had about had it with years of waiting for her husband to complete his training while she skimped and did without things that the other young women around her had. Also, there were the long, lonely hours and the husband who spent his infrequent time at home studying.

It's hard to be always on top in such circumstances. The husband, while he may be working and studying around the clock, nevertheless has the stimulation and the challenge of what he's involved with. All too often his wife has little relief from mere routine—and some get terribly depressed. I'm glad the Lord can use me to be a buffer, a sounding board, and I trust, an encouragement to these young women.

I learned too that being a doctor's wife is one thing; being the wife of an avowed *Christian* doctor is something else.

"You might as well get used to drinking and to serving liquor," I was informed by the more knowing wives. "It's the expected thing." Ralph was hearing the same: "In our circles everybody serves drinks at any social function and in the home." We settled this once and for all in our home. There would be no drinks. We have entertained literally thousands, both Christians and non-

Christians; never have we felt that anyone had less of a good time because of the absence of *the bottle.*

I remembered how my mother had handled the question in our home. Dad had come back from a trip east, and he said to Mother, "The girls [my sister and I] should learn to take a drink or two; all the young ladies are doing this, and I wouldn't want our two to be social misfits."

My mother was a strong Christian. "Over my dead body" was her response to Dad's suggestion. So drinking has never been a question in the Byron home.

Sometimes, people who know Ralph's public life ask me "What is he like at home?" On occasion a member of his King's Couples Sunday school class asks this, and I readily answer "Come home with me and you'll find out." Ralph is not two persons, one for the public and another for his family. Not for a minute! He doesn't have two faces. He's direct—almost to the point of bluntness at times, and basically his is a one-track mind. Although he has a wide variety of interests, his mind is totally engrossed with what he is doing at the moment.

What is my husband like at home? Well, for one thing, he doesn't bring the hospital home with him. He leaves his work; he doesn't ask us to carry his patient load. Oh, we're all interested in the great things that go on at the City of Hope: one of our sons and our son-in-law are doctors. But Ralph is wise enough to recognize that he can't live with pain and trauma every hour of his life and still remain objective and effective as a responsible surgeon.

Ralph is a very confident person. I might go so far as to say he has a big ego. As an only child and grandchild, his parents and his grandmother worked at making him feel important. This resulted in his having a very healthy image of himself and his abilities. Because of this, he is great at instilling confidence in other people. He can always find something positive to say about —and to—another person.

He's easy to live with. Like all of us, he has his faults. For one thing, he's messy; he leaves his belongings lying around. I scream. He laughs—and then we laugh together. He just steps out of his surgical garb at the hospital, and a nurse is there to pick up after him and the other doctors; he does the same at home. But he's the greatest person to live with; he lives and lets us live. And what a worker he is! You would have to hear the family tell about him and his backyard. He mows the grass himself, usually on Saturdays, and true to character, he scatters grass cuttings all over when he comes in the house. But we love him anyway.

Since people know Dr. Byron as a disciplined Bible student and memorizer of God's Word, and they've heard of his early morning vigil with God, I'm sometimes asked "How much of his high level dedication does he demand of the family and you, Mrs. Byron? Does he impose his standards on the rest of you? Does he expect you all to be up at dawn memorizing Bible verses?"

I can honestly say no to such questions. Certainly it's a tremendous heritage for children to grow up with such an example of a disciplined, dedicated life, but Ralph lets them live their own lives before the Lord. His influence on them is the result of love.

"What makes him maintain this schedule?" I'm sometimes asked, and usually the person will add, "We all have made similar vows to the Lord. But with most of us, these don't last. Doc keeps at it." I can only answer, that's the kind of person he is.

It has been a joy to me as I've thought how the Lord let Ralph and me meet when we did. Although he had been a Christian for a few years, he had been mainly marking time. When we started to go together I had known the Lord for only six months. So in a real sense, we've grown spiritually together. There has always been a unity of purpose in whatever either of us wanted to do for God, in our missionary giving or whatever kind of service the Lord had for us. Not that we haven't had differences of opinion; we have, but we've worked them out together. Between ourselves, or when the children have been involved, we have never let our differences become divisive.

Ralph is an idea person, and he can be very persuasive when he has a brainstorm. He's also such an inveterate optimist that (if you'll pardon the pun) he's the greatest for giving other people a shot in the arm when they most need it.

"He tends to play God," someone once said of my husband. The remark concerned his conviction that if he learns of a need that he can meet, he moves in with help. Maybe this is "playing

God." It has gotten him into some spots, especially when he has willingly loaned money to keep a fellow Christian out of trouble, more than once. For payment he has had to settle for the lesson it taught him. Nevertheless, the Scripture says, "Bear ye one another's burdens, and so fulfil the law of Christ" (Galatians 6:2). It's not enough to be able to quote the verse—especially when someone is in trouble. Would not this fall into the category of *standing in the gap?*

I've heard it said that in every successful doctor and particularly surgeons, there is a trace of the omnipotent, or at least a bid for it. Although it may be true, the surgeon I know best is humble even while he is confident; he knows God has given him a special place, and he strives to glorify God in that place.

Earlier my husband shared the decision I made when he asked me to marry him. I had to earnestly pray about it for I loved singing. My mother was a voice teacher, and although she would have enjoyed seeing me succeed in the opera world where fine doors were opening to me, it was Mother who helped me the most to find God's will at that crossroads in my life. She was very wise, and I saw that giving up the opera didn't mean I wouldn't sing at all. I concluded that God had given me this talent, and it was He who had brought Ralph and me together, and that my singing would be part of our life together. And it is. Ralph is so proud of my singing. People often say to me, "You should just see your husband when you're singing."

That's another thing about Ralph. He treats me like a queen. I hear him tell the fellows in his King's Couples class and other men's groups to "treat your wife like a queen." Sometimes I wonder if they know what he means. I do. He has me way up on a pedestal, and he always insists that the children treat me with the greatest respect. I suspect that his own dad was like that with his mother, and it rubbed off on Ralph.

Also my husband delights in bringing me presents from all the places he goes. He can't resist a bargain, and as a result, I have among a variety of other things, a pure silk dress from France, the kind that will never wear out and stays in style. I have china ornaments from here and there and a gorgeous silver service. Oh, let me tell you about that gift. Ralph was ready to come home from a midwest engagement when he spotted a gift shop. He crossed over to it intending to buy me a silver spoon. Well, he thought that wasn't much; he would buy a fine serving piece. Then he noticed a beautifully engraved serving tray. That's it, he decided. From there it was a short step for the salesperson to convince him there should be *something on the tray*. He ended up with a coffee server—the kind with an on-off spout—a teapot, a hot water pot, and the sugar and creamer. He arrived home about five in the morning. One of the children had been croupy, and I had just fallen asleep when he came, enthusiastic as always, and presented this impressive gift. Through the years I've enjoyed it, used it, and shown it off with pride. I treasure it, not only for its beauty and worth, but for the love that it represents. That early morning, in my half-asleep state, I know my response must have been disappointing to my husband.

I also proudly display a collection of toby jugs, the gift of our son Jon. His father's beautiful habit rubbed off on him.

Another of the treasures around our home is Ralph's journal (so this isn't his first book!). Besides his dedicated parents, Ralph, as a boy, had other encouragers. For instance, when he was about to go on a European tour at age twelve, he was given a notebook with one hundred pages and inscribed in it was:

> The purpose of these notes ought to be to make you accurate. If you write your thoughts down, and then in after years compare what you thought with your new thoughts, they will be very interesting. And it will help you to state things *just as they are*, not as your memory pictures them.
>
> It is better that you think wrong, *if you do your own thinking*, than to think right, and allow somebody to do your thinking for you.
>
> So write your thoughts down just as they come to you. There are one hundred pages in this book—one page for every day.

The unnamed friend surely must have been a teacher for it continues:

> This notebook is a present from a friend who wants you to learn to think straight.

I've smiled to myself from time to time as I've picked up this thick journal, most of it written in pencil in large, sprawling schoolboy style. The title page reads:

The
Travelogue
by
Ralph Byron, Jr.

Published by
Himself
1926

and the preface reads:

Being an accurate record
of the things he
SAW,
HEARD,
and
THOUGHT ABOUT
on a journey through Norway, Sweden,
and other countries during the summer
of nineteen twenty six.

Actually the journal covered many countries that Ralph was privileged to tour; he recorded something about them all. Spelling was not his great subject; so he saw in the House of Lords where the *dilegates* sit; in Ireland, he wrote of seeing *Pete* bogs; in Egypt, *Mumies;* in Jerusalem, a *Mosk*. Later, the friend who gave Ralph the notebook and thus started him writing, advised that he present his endeavors to a person who would objectively critique it and then help him correct the spelling.

There is so much in this journal. A later trip to the Mediterranean countries sparked this observation: "The funny thing about the sports deck is that there are enclosed seats for two—and no young people on board . . . there are innumerable little hideouts for two . . . ."

Two things stand out to me as I think about Ralph's journal:

one, that he recognized and respected the intent of the friend who offered the notebook with his counsel; two, that having started to make a record, Ralph diligently kept it up, never missing one day. I think of all the things on such trips that would have kept me from sticking with a diary but *this is Ralph!* He finishes what he starts. Also, he was most precise about such things as the ship's tonnage, the height of the mountains he saw, and the historical facts and figures. I feel that in the journal of the boy there is revealed the character of the man I married. It is proved more each day.

It's a humbling experience to be the wife of such a man. I'm no women's libber. I firmly believe in the biblical concept of love and lordship, a picture of Christ and His church. This is the essence of marriage; this is the happy marriage. Ralph and I have proved this together, and it has been thirty-five super years.

Why the *little corporal?* That's how Ralph speaks of me. Maybe it's because I'm a little bossy; maybe it's to remind him of his important years in the marines. Somebody asked him one day "Why do you call Dorothy a corporal? Why not a higher rank?"

"Well," he said with that enigmatic smile of his, "when you're just a private [meaning himself], a corporal is somebody to be reckoned with." Whatever his reason, people who know us always knew who Ralph means when he speaks of the *little corporal.*

12 Up the Ladder—and *Down*

For many people the climb up the ladder of success is long, hard, and slow. In the providence of God, this was not my experience. Things seemed to fall my way; doors of opportunity appeared to have my name on them. Everything was rosy—while it lasted.

When I finished my training period (my wife thought it would never end), I had to decide where to practice. One doesn't have unlimited options, but is governed by the available opportunities. I was no exception to this. There was the possibility of opening an office in Berkeley where I would be near my very good friend Robert B. Munger and his church. Here I would have a *solo* surgical practice. This would be difficult at the beginning but would ultimately be satisfactory.

In Napa, a small California city, the surgeon of the leading medical combine had suddenly died. I was asked to go look over the setup. I did, but somehow it did not seem to be the type of practice which would use my training or provide opportunities for me to serve the Lord.

One of the young established surgeons in San Francisco asked me to go in with him as a partner. This had a certain attractiveness; he had a good practice, reputation, and best of all, was easy to work with. While I was considering this, a new possibility came on the horizon.

The telephone rang. I answered it, and heard my former professor's voice, "I have a great opportunity at the university [University of California Medical School, San Francisco] for you. Come over and I'll explain it to you." I took off immediately, roared over to the medical school, and went to the professor's office. He told me in glowing terms what he had for me; a cancer institute was being set up at the school, and I would be the assistant director. (There would be no director for a time.) I would be an instructor in the surgery department with a salary, teaching opportunities, and research facilities. I would be allowed to do private surgery to supplement my income. It was a dream setup! I prayed about it with my wife, and it seemed obvious that this was a God-given opportunity. I grabbed it and told the Lord, perhaps impetuously, I would *never* leave, and if He ever wanted me to depart from the university fold, He would have to have them throw me out! Time would prove God's faithfulness to me in meeting my conditions.

My time at the university was a delight. I was a fair-haired boy and could do no wrong. For the first time in my life I had a secretary. I didn't know what to do with her, but I had her. I even had a second secretary to help the first. I didn't know what to do with her either. Surgical cases were referred to me. They were big surgical procedures with real challenges. Little did I know that they were being sent to me, not because of my ability, but because I represented the university. In research I worked with Dr. B., who was brilliant, talented, and loaded with ideas. He did the medical aspects, and I did the surgery. We hit it off like a hand in a glove. Our work was beginning to be published regularly. My reputation was growing.

My opportunities to serve the Lord were numerous. My time was my own except for the few assignments at the medical school. I ran the tumor board, which is a once-a-week consultation by surgeons to discuss and determine procedure regarding difficult and unusual cancer cases. As chairman, this was a valuable experience, and helped me in dealing with the administrators of the hospital.

If the question arose in my mind, "Lord, what about that verse You gave me? When is that going to be activated in my life, a distinct ministry to Your chosen people?" I could silence the mild unrest. This must be God's will for me for the present. Hadn't He made the opening for me?

I had a large Bible class on Sundays, numerous speaking engagements, and assignments in the church, such as an elder and chairman of the missions department. My income had increased dramatically, and so did my giving. Dorothy and I undertook to put three students through school, help in the support of a missionary couple, and give generously to the church. This amounted to one-third of our gross income. Things were going smoothly.

As I indicated, when I came to the university I had fallen heir to a great secretary. She was everything a secretary should be, loyal, talented, dependable, and a perfectionist about her work. I was naive enough to think all secretaries were like this. When an opportunity came for her to take a better position, I gladly released her. As I looked for a new secretary, I again had fortune smile on me in the form of a brilliant, talented, Jewish girl. She was having marital problems and had decided to work for a while.

After being with me for a time, she asked me, "What do Christians think of Jews?" I told her how God had used the Jew; took her through the Old Testament, told her of the prophecies of the Messiah, and showed her the fulfillment in the New Testament in Christ. We discussed this further, almost daily. One day I said, "Myra, would you like to accept Christ as your Lord and personal Savior?" She was taken aback. Up to this point, it had been like a briefing. All of a sudden, it had become very, very personal. She said, "Will you give me twenty-four hours to give you an answer?" I answered, "Sure." The next morning she came to me and said, "The answer is no! The price is too high! I would lose my husband, my family, and my friends. I would have no one." We continued to talk about the Gospel in the days that followed. Then one morning she came to me and said, "I can't talk about Christ anymore; I can't sleep at night!" I answered, "Very well, I won't say anything unless you introduce the subject." The next day I was to speak to a luncheon put on in Berkeley for the Inter-Varsity students. I said, "Myra, how would you like to go with me to the meeting?"

"I'd love to," she answered. "I love going to meetings."

"This will be a spiritual meeting," I warned her.

"I don't care what kind it is; I like meetings," she insisted.

We took off for the Inter-Varsity meeting; Myra was in high spirits.

I spoke from an Old Testament passage as I presented the

Gospel. She listened but appeared unmoved. I closed with prayer then went to her table to get her for the return trip. She was totally speechless, most uncharacteristic of her.

"What's the matter?" I asked. I will never forget her response.

"That is the very first time I ever heard anyone really pray."

There was total silence on the way back. Then two days later she said, "You've ruined it for me. Now I will *never* accept Christ."

I thought, *What have I done? How have I failed the Lord?* I searched my heart. I was crushed as I sought to relive the preceding hours. All I said to Myra was, "I don't know what I've done to make you feel the way you do, but whatever it was, you've learned a most important lesson."

"Oh—*what?*" she asked.

"If you keep your eyes on me, as a Christian, sooner or later, you will be disappointed; but if you keep your eyes on Christ, you will never be disappointed."

Three days later she came to me and dramatically said, "I've just accepted Christ as my Savior!"

All I could blurt out was, "Tell me about it." And she did.

"I was in the Safeway Market," she began, "over by the fresh vegetables [she said this as though it was all-important which part of the store she had been in] and I thought *this is as good a place as any for me to do this*. So I bowed my head and invited Christ to come into my heart as Lord and Savior."

"Great!" I applauded her action. Then I could not resist asking her what she had meant by saying I had "ruined it" for her. Her reply to that was, "I knew even then that I was going to accept Christ; I just didn't want you to know."

Following this experience, three things happened in rapid succession that were to change my life. First, the professor of surgery called me in with a thinly veiled complaint. "When my wife and I came to this university," he began, "we did not drink. However, we soon learned that around these circles one has to drink and to serve drinks in his home. We accommodated to this, Doctor—and I suggest you do the same."

My response to this was, "You are a great surgeon and have taught me a lot, but my wife and I do not drink, and we do not serve alcohol in our home. When people come to our house, we feed them well, and try to see that they have a good time, but we insist they play it our way." Needless to say, this went over like a lead balloon.

The second piece on the chessboard of my life at that time was a potential great stride forward. The university was about to appoint a full director of the cancer research institute. All unknown to me, I was the front-runner for the position. However, because of a series of misunderstandings, the department heads did not think I was eager to accept the position. It was then that wheels that put me out of the medical school forever began to turn.

I had made it clear to the Lord that I would never leave of my own accord. Then a third incident involving a disloyal secretary clinched it.

Like an atomic bomb going off, the word reached me that my stay at the medical school was to be terminated. Everything came to an end at once: my salary, my office, my secretary, my patient referrals, and all the reputation that I accrued by being at the university. I had to find an office; I had to start over; I had to begin again. I rented space in a nearly finished medical building, but a carpenters' strike delayed its completion for five months. I didn't even have a home base. Even my old patients couldn't find me. I was hitting bottom.

13 God's Clock Strikes

In the days following the medical school fiasco, I wondered whether God would dramatically step in and rescue us from the evil that had befallen us; but He didn't.

It was immediately apparent that I was in a completely new ball game. What a shock to learn that it was not the magic of my name that had drawn patients, but the reputation of the university. Also, while I had of course heard surgeons talk about the overhead and expenses of a private practice, now suddenly, I was in the midst of it all. It was a road I had not traveled before.

During the four years since my training ended, money had come to me with comparative ease. Now, here I was with three growing children whose needs and wants grew at least as quickly as they did. At the same time my income dropped at an alarming rate. Another grave concern was our missionary and church commitments. Should we write the people concerned and explain our situation and that we regretfully could no longer support them?

The only buffer we had at the start of this period was $1600 in the bank. Could we possibly continue to give away $550 a month in our bleak financial crisis?

We prayed about this, discussing it with God: "Lord, what do *You* want us to do? Wouldn't You understand if we go back on our pledges? Certainly You know we cannot give what we don't have." It was a spiritual crisis on the down-where-we-live, practical level, the nitty-gritty of the Christian walk.

As we prayed and reasoned, God brought to my remembrance an Old Testament story. It was from the life of the Prophet Elijah (*see* 1 Kings 17:1–16). God had instructed Elijah to warn a wicked king, Ahab, that it wouldn't rain for three and one-half years. Elijah then had to flee from the king's wrath, and the Lord caused ravens to feed him when he was at the brook Cherith. This was extraordinary, since the raven is a scavenger bird. The brook dried up and God directed Elijah to a place called Zarephath and told him a *widow* would feed him (again, an unlikely source). Though at first unwilling to share the little she had for herself and her son, she listened to Elijah when he said, "Give me, the man of God, a little first, and you have God's promise that the barrel of meal shall not waste, neither shall the cruse of oil fail, until the day that the Lord sendeth rain upon the earth" (1 Kings 17:14). The widow did as Elijah requested, and true to God's promise, she had enough for herself and her son until the drought ended.

We, my wife, our three children, and I, were in the midst of drought. There was no question about that! As I prayerfully considered what God was directing my thoughts to, I knew He was saying to me, "Keep up your commitments to Me, and I will take care of you." What a challenge! We accepted it; we did keep those commitments, somehow. We started with that $1600 bank account, went through three and one-half unbelievably difficult years, met every commitment we had made to the Lord, and—wonder of wonders—at the end of that period we had $1600 in the bank!

In our society we are so money oriented that there's a tendency to feel that if we have to struggle financially we must be off the track. Actually there is very little truth in that. The thing to watch for is the spiritual blessing or lack of it. I can honestly say that there have been few times in my life when God was pleased to bless me more than during that drought. He even graciously worked it so that no one knew how much we were struggling with our finances. I'm here to testify that we had everything we needed—and much, much more.

One of the real delights was that the Lord had opened the way for a home Bible class, a once-a-month dinner meeting in Orinda where we had our home. It was a bring-your-own-food, rotate-from-house-to-house gathering. We called them Bible reading classes. Because even the largest of the homes could accommodate a maximum of seventy-five people, that had to be our limit.

Then I invited a patient and her husband to attend. This woman was so enthused that she wanted to start a similar class in their home. She, Betty Stokes, was the world's best saleswoman when it came to drumming up interest in this new Bible class. We began in September with eighty-five present; by Christmas there were three hundred. As you must have guessed, it was a spacious home (in the Hillsborough area of Patty Hearst fame). As the numbers grew the class caught the interest of the media, and a reporter from the *Oakland Tribune* did a photo story spread for the Sunday *Parade* section of June 12, 1955.

Orinda doctor leads a crusade

Healing souls and bodies

By BILL ROSE
Tribune church editor

One day 12 years ago, in 1943, Dr. Ralph Byron was reading his Bible in his Orinda home. In the 23rd chapter of Ezekiel he read verse 30, and paused. He reread it.

"And I sought for a man among them, that should make up the hedge, and *stand in the gap* before me for the land, that I should not destroy it. . ."

At that moment, Dr. Byron, a cancer specialist, determined to "stand in the gap" and devote his energies to healing souls as well as bodies.

From that decision several important events stemmed, two of them notable: the organization of the Orinda-Lafayette Presbyterian Church, and the organization of a Bible study class drawing residents of the Bay Area to a smart Peninsula home each month.

It was shortly after his decision was made that Dr. Byron closed his San Francisco office and joined the Marines as a medical officer. In his two years of service in the South Pacific he organized Bible classes among the leathernecks when they gathered early for the weekly movie. At first he was received rather coolly, but his

> audiences later warmed up and he achieved quite a success in his unusual venture.
>
> Returned from overseas, he reopened his offices and formed a Bible study group among his Orinda neighbors. The group expanded quickly and vigorously and some of the more enthusiastic members became enthused with the idea of organizing a church. Thus did the Orinda-Lafayette Presbyterian Church come into being.
>
> About two years ago Dr. Byron invited one of his patients, Mrs. Ralph Stokes of Hillsborough, to attend his Bible study class. She accepted and was fired with zeal to extend the work. With her husband's help, she established a Bible study group which meets two nights each month in their 28-room Hillsborough home (it once was rented to the former Barbara Hutton for a six-month period).
>
> Dr. Byron agreed to help out, reading and explaining Bible passages at the meetings, the first of which attracted 80 people. Now each meeting attracts 250 to 300 people and the first year anniversary was attended by 750. More than 2,000 individuals have attended.
>
> As the movement grew the leaders were joined by Arnold Grunegan, a stocks and bonds man, and Ted Atkinson, an office manager, both of San Francisco.
>
> The Bible sessions are genial affairs. Children of the members are sent to upstairs quarters where a trained nurse puts the younger ones to bed and tells a biblical story to the older ones. Downstairs, the hosts having welcomed their guests at the door, Dr. Byron, using no notes, interprets the Bible stories. The meeting over, coffee and tea are served and a snack is eaten; the guests bring their own food.
>
> The meetings are anything but solemn and stiff affairs. On this occasion [when the reporter was present] Mrs. Byron sang.

My wife's lovely voice was a great asset, and the Holy Spirit was able to use her singing of beautiful Gospel hymns to set the climate for listening to God's Word. Also, Dorothy's warm, outgoing personality and her *joy* in being a Christian couldn't help but impress these people. Meeting after meeting, decisions were made for Christ, and lives changed.

It was gratifying to know that the Lord was using Dorothy and me in this strategic ministry. I say strategic because, all too often, little attention is paid to the spiritual needs of the people who are wealthy in the material sense. Perhaps this is what Jesus had in mind when He stated, "How hard it is for the rich to enter the kingdom of God!" (Matthew 19:23 NIV). Many rich persons never hear a direct presentation of the Gospel or learn of their own need to make sure they spend eternity with Christ.

I know many who are *churchmen* but who are being systematically robbed of the direct preaching and teaching that "all have sinned, and come short of the glory of God" (Romans 3:23) and "the wages of sin is death; but the gift of God is eternal life through Jesus Christ our Lord" (Romans 6:23).

So I have always been grateful to the Lord for the privilege He gave me to present the simple, direct Word of God in Hillsborough to that group that included wealthy socialites. Their spiritual needs are as great—often greater—than less affluent listeners.

Because of the cosmopolitan nature of the San Francisco area, we had the privilege of having at least one person from almost every country in the world present at those Bible classes. In a sense we were fulfilling Christ's commission to go into all the world and preach the Gospel. Nevertheless, never too far from the surface was that definite commission I had felt from the Lord that day sitting in a foreign airport. Oh, don't get me wrong. I don't mean that I felt the present wasn't important. I've never had that idea. Each day is important for what opportunities it holds to live and serve and learn that day. But that verse, Ezekiel 3:5, had been so real:

> For thou are not sent to a people of a strange speech . . . but to the house of Israel.

Had God forgotten? Had I attached too great significance to this call? Was I not yet ready in God's eyes for this assignment?

God's clock was about to strike. It was evident to me that God used particular individuals, not only in Bible times, but also in leading people in our own time. In my life I had ample evidence of this as one step led to another.

While I was in practice in San Francisco, God began to set wheels in motion to activate His plan according to the verse He had given me. One of my good friends with whom I worked at the University of California had joined the staff of the City of Hope. We had done research and patient care together, and he, Dr. H.B., was instrumental in having me invited to the City of Hope.

But, you may recall from an earlier chapter, this medical center was committed to its purpose as a tuberculosis sanatorium. Where would I fit into their program?

Oh, but things had changed from that era when buildings replaced the original two tents in the desert for the care of victims of the dread disease. In the forties it appeared that tuberculosis might become a conquered disease; that would have put the City of Hope out of business. The board of directors wrestled with this and decided that their challenge was the *catastrophic nature* of tuberculosis. Why not then, include other catastrophic diseases: cancer, leukemia, heart disease, and diabetes. The metamorphosis was beginning to take place when I first laid eyes on the City of Hope.

That was December, 1953—and it didn't look too *hopeful,* as I saw the approach of unkept grounds and weeds. It was a disaster! However, as we neared the main buildings, there were trim lawns, trees, and flowers. I made my own observation, and the administration looked at me and my credentials that time, then again in 1954, and in early 1955.

On August 2 that year—ten years *to the day* from the time God had given me His assignment—it was literally fulfilled when I was appointed chief of surgery at the City of Hope.

I felt it; I knew it, that all the preparation God had been putting me through and all the lessons He had been teaching me were for this, my lifework. About that time I had been reading and studying God's dealings with Abraham. I had just read where God told him to "Arise, walk through the land in the length of it and in the breadth of it; for I will give it unto thee" (Genesis 13:17).

Never a person to do things halfway, I figured I'd better walk over the whole City of Hope premises, ninety-two acres. Hour after hour as I crisscrossed those acres, I'm sure there were many doctors wondering what that nutty surgeon was doing, walking in the wilds of nowhere.

Oh, but none of them had waited ten years to find this place!

14 The End of the Quest

How can I ever fully articulate what it meant to me the day I officially became a part of the City of Hope? There were ten years of pondering and dreaming and wondering and speculating *Just what is it You have in mind for me, God? Where* are *these, the "house of Israel," You have so impressed on my mind and heart?*

Here I was, at the very heart of one of the greatest single examples of Jewish humanitarian endeavor in all the world!

For us, accepting a position at the City of Hope, was a returning home to Los Angeles—a full cycle. It had taken the experiences of the years away, and the people whose lives had touched mine to help make needed changes. Most of all, we had learned what God can and does do for us when we believe Him. It doesn't always take so long. God apparently can shape some men and women in just a few years.

The City of Hope had grown, unbelievably, from that first compassionate dedication to *do something* for the hopeless victims of tuberculosis. Through the years, women's auxiliaries have been formed in almost every state, and their zeal and heartfelt interest accounts for an impressive part of the annual income. Not only a fund-raising institution, these auxiliary women carry on an education program, similar to the American Cancer Society.

The personnel that the City of Hope attracts includes some of the brightest young researchers in the world. They come, and as our astronauts said of themselves, "stand on the shoulders of the giants who preceded them" to carry on relentless research that will effectively war on catastrophic diseases.

Bright, highly motivated MDs, both men and women, vie to take additional training at the City of Hope. This is my specialty, and one of the greatest joys of my life is to work with and to train in surgery such potential-loaded men and women. It's one of the highlights of each year for my wife and me when we invite them from wherever they are under God's heaven to come for a barbecue and a reunion at our home. Such times we have then! Interestingly, laced into the conversation I hear snatches of the quotes and sayings for which I've come to be known. God knows I have prayed for each and have witnessed to them. It's a good feeling now to hear, among the reminiscences of the riotous fun things we shared—and believe me, we laughed a lot—that these other eternal truths have stuck with them. I should say that it came to me that when one of my associates was asked "What's it like working with Dr. Byron?" the quick answer was "He's a riot!" Well, why not? Why shouldn't a happy man project some of his mirth? It's a dreary world for most people, and nothing is more true in the whole Bible than "A merry heart doeth good like a medicine" (Proverbs 17:22). As a Christian *and a doctor,* I believe in this prescription. And I like to practice it which brings to mind a story.

A stranger came to town and inquired of a resident "Where does Dr. Smith live?" "Which Dr. Smith?" the person asked. "We have two, the one who *preaches* and the one who *practices."* I like to think God lets me do both. It's my constant prayer that there be no bridge between what I believe and how I perform.

As a Christian I can't compartmentalize my life. It's not a matter of a Christian having Sunday things, words, and feelings for when we're with our fellow believers, and a set that's different for our everyday world. There would have to be a great lack of integrity in such ambivalence. Such could never be God's intent for the Bible says, "whatsoever ye do, do it heartily, as to the Lord" (Colossians 3:23). What we think, is ultimately lived out in our lives.

Running as parallel as a set of railroad tracks must be the work I do and the words I quote. I must never let myself become satisfied with anything less than the pursuit of excellence. This reminds me of a surgeon whom I admire, Dr. Viggo Olsen of Bangladesh. When in the course of his searching he felt God's call to serve Him on the mission field, this was the doctor's heartfelt response. "If I am going to represent Jesus Christ as a surgeon in a foreign country, then I must be at least as good as the best surgeon they have in that country." He proceeded to make sure he would pass his own test. This is the pursuit of excellence.

When with God's help we can be this kind of person, it can have dual results. One, we can have a positive impact on those around us, and secondly, we can help open doors of opportunity for other people who are eager to witness for the Lord.

My good friend Dr. Clyde Narramore was on a plane going east, and in conversation with his fellow passenger, learned that she was a doctor and that she was returning from a medical conference at the City of Hope. "Oh, I know one of the surgeons there," he said, and mentioned my name.

"Dr. Byron? Yes, I've met him. He's very religious." After a pause she added, "He also knows what he's doing."

It was gratifying to me when Dr. Narramore relayed this to me. But I found myself wondering if like myself in my earlier days, this doctor had a hard time equating being religious with any high goals in one's profession. What a paradox! The very One we profess to be following "did all things well." I was glad my name had not been a stumbling block.

A move inevitably means looking, not only for a new home, but a new church home. At the time, Dr. Halverson, assistant minister of Hollywood Presbyterian Church, was just leaving, and I was invited to replace him as teacher of a large Sunday school class. Soon we were involved with the Voyager Class there. But while we loved the church and the pastor and everything about *Hollywood Pres,* it was just too far for the family, if we were to be a part of all the activities. This led us to a church in nearby Pasadena, the Lake Avenue Congregational Church. It had what we wanted in a church, a clear-cut presentation of the Gospel with an opportunity for individuals to face up to their need of Christ as Savior and Lord. We saw a group of enthusiastic, warmhearted believers, and the missionary outreach was impressive. In 1957 I was invited to become the teacher of a Sunday school class named the King's Couples. Dorothy and I agreed, but only on condition that we could be a real part of the class. They agreed to that, and for a couple of years I carried on both classes, dashing on Sunday mornings between Pasadena and Hollywood.

The days went by bringing great gratification to me. Here I was where *God* had placed me, doing what I loved to do. Spiritually, there were many opportunities; professionally, my life was both rewarding and exciting. Then, in a way I could never even have dreamed of, suddenly my position at the City of Hope was in jeopardy.

I came to the City of Hope because of one man, Dr. H.B. We had worked together at the University of California and had become great friends. After coming to the City of Hope in 1953, he did all the groundwork to arrange for me to follow him two years later when we were reunited and continued our research and patient care together. A scant three years after I had arrived at the City of Hope, Dr. H.B. got into difficulty with the board of directors and was terminated. Because of my close association with this doctor, it was a foregone conclusion that I would go also. However, I was in no way connected with his difficulties. Moreover, I was at the City of Hope because I felt this was where God wanted me.

What a dilemma! Would God intervene, and if so, how was He going to accomplish it? I prayed more fervently than ever.

The key doctor at the hospital, Dr. M.J., had taken it for granted that I was on the way out. It was he whom God tapped on the shoulder at this time of crisis in my life. A rather unusual episode triggered it. At the time, a little twelve-year-old girl was dying of cancer in Beverly Hills. The parents were anxious that their daughter not know of her true condition. Fearing that going to the City of Hope would spell doom for her—that she would guess her diagnosis—they requested that two consultants come from the City of Hope to see her in her home. Dr. M.J. and I were the ones asked to go and I asked him to ride with me. He agreed.

We rode the fifty or so miles to the strange, poignant rendezvous. We met the grief-stricken parents, saw the little girl, made our pronouncements, and dropped our *words of wisdom* (*so inade-*

quate, I realized then and do now). Then we started back to the hospital.

It was on that ride back that Dr. M.J. and I shared our objectives. No doubt our feelings of frustration at being helpless to save this child's life gnawed at us and drew us together. As we talked of our goals for the City of Hope and our patients, we discovered that we were on the same track—the pursuit of excellence, nothing else and nothing less. This was God's specific answer to my prayer; any threat to my position at the City of Hope was then and there dispelled. That was the beginning of a friendship that has remained, since we are close associates at the hospital. God had worked everything out just right. That was nineteen years ago.

At the City of Hope the concerns of the patient and his family are not lost on us. We care beyond the scope of the disease. We are not peddling health on the hoof. We are conscious of the needs of the whole, the total person. Because it's hard for a patient either to face surgery, or to recuperate following it if his mind is focused on the family problems caused by his hospitalization, we have programs designed to alleviate such anxiety. In this, the City of Hope is ahead of its time. In a *Los Angeles Times* article titled "Cancer Families Learn to Cope," the writer quoted Stanford University Professor Dr. David M. Kaplan as saying:

> . . . professionals who treat cancer patients are beginning to grapple with the psycho-social problems suffered by cancer patients and their families.

At the City of Hope, no effort is ever made to recruit any material support from the patient. On the contrary, every effort is made to discourage him from thinking about money. But cured of his illness, and sent back into the world with his self-respect intact, many a patient has become imbued with the ideology he had seen in practice by every level of the staff. It is constantly affirmed and reiterated that the patient owes no debt to the City of Hope. There are varying reactions to this. One patient voiced her hesitation about becoming what she called a charity case, but she changed her thinking when her doctor pointed out to her that she was making a great contribution by permitting herself to be operated on (she had a rare form of cancer).

Others, while not feeling they are in any way obligated because of the help they received, nevertheless, out of sheer gratitude, want to share and to do something to pass it on. The letter from such a patient reads:

> I came to the City of Hope in 1955 with no hope for my life of any kind. Your doctors told me at that time to go back home and wait . . . On July 9, 1957 I was called back to the City of Hope and your staff performed one of your first open heart operations on me. From July 11 of that year until now, I have lived—and I mean I have really lived. Life is so wonderful because I am now able to do just a little for others. This is my way of trying to say thank you.

Even when in spite of all that we could do the patient died, the relatives have sometimes taken up the cause. No where is this more true than in the heartbreak of children with leukemia.

Hope lives on. One of these days all the faith, all the dedicated research, will pay off; another enemy of the human body will be defeated. Meanwhile, we plug away at what the Lord gives us to do, feeling that each day's work is good for its own sake, and marveling at the way He has led us until this day. My own experience reminds me of the verse, "A man's heart deviseth his way: but the LORD directeth his steps" (Proverbs 16:9).

I might have schemed and planned and manipulated toward a certain goal, *devising my way;* thank God He showed me early in my Christian walk that He had a step at a time for me, and that He was directing my path. God always knew that the end of my quest would be the City of Hope.

I've pondered many times, the specific things God ploughs into us, as preparation for what He has for us to do. The pursuit of excellence was a goal the Lord would never let me compromise. There came the day in the fifties when the City of Hope, under the magnificent leadership of its president, Dr. Ben Horowitz, expanded its horizons. While retaining all its compassionate patient care for the victims of catastrophic diseases, it branched out as a pilot medical center to influence science and medicine everywhere. Significantly, among the decisions governing this monumental change was this as Levenstein noted:

> . . . A new type of staff would have to be assembled, chosen on the basis of creativity and committed to the pursuit of excellence.

15 What Our Children Can Teach Us

You may be wondering why there hasn't been much said about the younger Byrons. Well, it would take a book to tell just about them.

I learned some of my greatest lessons in living from my children. As an only child, I had missed out on what must surely be invaluable experiences, the adjustments and the daily give-and-take of growing up with a family of brothers and sisters. What books (with the exception of the Book of Proverbs) could possibly offer such insight and understanding of how to cope with a world of other people?

To me in my inexperience, even the simple, little emergencies assumed great proportions—until I began to learn about such things. Perhaps the greatest single thing my children taught me about human nature is that *no two persons are alike.* A great discovery!

Joanne was about four and one-half when her brother, Rod, came to bless our home. A blessing he was and still is, but because we had not changed our minds one little bit about the importance of parents spending time with their children, we now had two children to take every place we went. Take them we did!

I found that it was very easy to transmit my interest in sports to Rod. He soaked up the statistics and was soon able to recite the batting average and record of teams and players, even the obscure ones. Sports became more important than school. Yes, you guessed it, he did poorly in school. If this wasn't bad enough, he developed a fear and a secret belief that he could never do well in school. Studying, which had been so easy for me, became a nightmare for him. This crept up on me, as I was confidently expecting him, like oil, to rise to the top in school. Actually, he was becoming mired more deeply in the mud.

To add to my woes, it became apparent that Joanne and Rod were being lost in our shadow. The measure of success that Dorothy and I had was hurting our children, and we didn't know it. On one hand, they were basking in the sunshine of our successes and our bragging about them, and on the other, they were developing an inner conviction that they could never attain what their parents had—so why try. They showed a if-I-don't-play-the-game-I-can't-lose attitude.

Rod, especially, suffered from these feelings. Rod is now an outstanding medical student although he considers himself a late bloomer. In later years, Joanne has confided her frustrations which affected her life, even after marriage, until one day she realized how very human and fallible her mother and I are.

For some reason, Dorothy was the first to sense the problem and had to relay it to me. I remember how totally flabbergasted I was. I could scarcely believe it, but it was only too true. I found myself driven to the Lord to ask forgiveness and to ask Him to give me insight and help in combating this evil. I've learned that the Lord is infinitely more interested in our children than we, as parents, ever could be, and His promise is "If any of you lack wisdom, [and I surely did] let him ask of God . . . and it shall be given him" (James 1:5).

Because of the nature of our problem, the first step very obviously was to quit using ourselves as examples: "This is the way I did it," and "Here's how your mother and I do it" had to become no-no's.

This reversal process took time, believe me; we had to bite our tongues a time or two. It was apparent to Dorothy and me that we would have to work long and hard to correct our course.

In time the Lord gave us another son, Jonathan; he too would teach us many things, but at least we had changed a little bit before we began to make our imprint on his life. Jon, like his sister and brothers, is blessed with his mother's vocal talent; he has a rich, baritone voice. He's the tall one, and he doesn't let us forget it. "I'm the only Byron over five feet ten inches; I can look down on Dad," he quips.

I frequently had heard that it's as easy to bring up two or three children as it is to raise just one. What a myth! Apart from everything else, my children taught me a new dimension in the field of medicine: if one caught a cold, they all caught a cold, and thoughtfully passed it back and forth. They even shared it with their parents. Nice, huh?

Another discovery I can attribute to Joanne, Rod, and Jon is that when sickness strikes, a doctor and his wife can be as panic-stricken as any of their lay friends who are parents.

Our fourth child, Rick, was born after we moved to southern California and I was at the City of Hope. We began to find that four children to care for is a full-time vocation. Rick was, as they say, all boy with a mind of his own, and he didn't hesitate to assert it. When he was about thirteen months old, I had just put him in his crib and left the room when he promptly climbed over the side rails and came toddling into the room with us. I quickly put him back to bed, and told him I would spank him if he got out again. Scarcely had I turned my back, when he was over the side rails. True to my word I spanked his little diapered behind, and told him that a repeat performance would result in a spanking with his pants down. Undaunted, he promptly got out of the crib. True to my word, I took his pants down, spanked him, and put him to bed, warning him that if he got out again, I would make him stand in the corner of the room. Without hesitation, he got over the side rails and onto the floor. I put him in the corner and stood guard. He turned his little head and looked up at me with a forlorn look. In my whole life I never felt like such a mean giant of a bully!

Rick would grow up to realize that dogged persistence can be a very fine quality, but not when, as in this instance, the persistence is linked to disobedience.

Each of the four resembles his parents in certain ways; yet they have qualities and abilities which far exceed those of their mother and father. Joanne meets problems head-on and drives a project to a successful conclusion, much as I do. She has her mother's warmth and spontaneity and an outgoing personality.

Rod, in his love for sports and statistics, is like me; he too, has the sensitivity that so marks his mother. Jon has a big heart for people, like his Mom, and a memory like mine. Rick is endowed with boundless energy and can do several things at once, like me. Since he is the one who is still at home, Rick is still teaching me a number of things.

Like other Christian parents, we have prayed much for our children's spiritual growth. It was almost immediately apparent that there was no super pill I could give them to guarantee that they would love God.

Each has learned to pray by saying his prayers at night with me. (The Bible is pretty specific about teaching your children "when they lie down" [*see* Deuteronomy 11:19], as well as other definite times; wherever possible, it seems to me, this is the *father's* duty and privilege.) They prayed, then they heard me pray. Somehow they grasped not only the importance of prayer, but how to pray.

I always made a practice of telling the children a story at bedtime. I chose Bible stories and in this way the children became familiar with most of the Bible in this *fun* way (the Bible has a never-ending assortment of thrillers, and children love to hear them over and over). Little by little our children came to love the Word of God as Dorothy and I do. Many of these lessons are *caught* rather than *taught*.

As we have done many things together as a family, the children, unbeknown to us, have been watching our every move. They have learned a little of how a husband should treat his wife, how to approach problems, how to win, how to lose, how to pick one's self up after failure, and most of all, the importance of having Christ first in one's life.

As parents, our own integrity (or lack of it) rubs off on our children; it is far more effective than all the lecturing we might do. Another thing I've learned is that some rules in surgery apply equally well in the lives of our children. For example, we have this rule in surgery: Good judgment comes from experience; experience comes from bad judgment. Sometimes we have to stand by and let our child make his own mistakes, if he is to gain the experience and the maturity that it seems can only come from bad judgment.

Ultimately, the lesson both Dorothy and I greatly needed was that we do not own our children. We can bring them into this world, love them, nurture them, and provide for their physical, emotional, and spiritual needs. But the time inevitably comes when having committed them to God's care, we willingly let them go. Only then can there be a continuing desirable relationship, as they live their own lives. How much heartache could be avoided if parents could just see this!

The fact is, we learn some of life's most important lessons from our children.

16 With Scalpel and Bible

Dr. Byron had been ten years at the City of Hope when the book, *Testimony for Man* was written. In a chapter titled, "The Men of the City," Levenstein wrote of Dr. Byron:

> One's first impression is that of a tall, grey man with troubled eyes that have seen much of death—both in World War II as a member of the Navy Medical Corps and in his lifelong war with the implacable enemy, cancer.
>
> Surgery, research and teaching have been the dominant interests of his professional life. He taught surgery at the University of California Medical School and was assistant director of its Cancer Research Institute. Professional associations and research centers constantly seek his counsel.
>
> But the tributes he has received from colleagues throughout the world bring him less satisfaction than the tribute he reads on the faces of City of Hope patients. Men, women and children who are on the way to the operating table or who are on the road back to recovery wait eagerly for his visits to their bedside and the opportunity to commune with him. From his prodigious reading and photographic memory, he gives them verbatim quotations to suit their moods and to hearten them in the fight for life. Their confidence in him comes not only from his reputation in his field but from the words with which he lifts their spirits.
>
> As a cancer specialist he has pioneered in the com-

bined use of surgery, radiology and drugs where each method by itself has not proved adequate. His scientific papers on new techniques in chemo-therapy, by which cancer-fighting drugs can be concentrated directly on tumors to minimize the hazard to healthy tissues, have sparked additional research by others.

In this age of skepticism Dr. Byron is a rare person. Even to some of his colleagues he is an anomaly—a scientific mind in the person of a "Biblical man." For Dr. Byron's is not only a life of science but a life of Biblical idealism. As philosopher Martin Buber has said: "The genuine life of faith develops on the spiritual heights, but it springs from the depths of the distress of the earth-bound body."

Few clergymen can match him in Bible scholarship. It has been said that if the Bible were destroyed, it could soon be reassembled from the memories of men who know whole chapters by heart; in such an event, Dr. Byron, a leading layman in the Congregational Church, would be one of the principal contributors. His conversation is laced with phrases from the King James version that come naturally to his lips. In response to a question about new "cures" for cancer published in the sensational popular press, he says, as if to himself: "I Corinthians 13," and then continues without faltering on a single syllable:

> Though I speak with the tongues of men and of angels, and have not charity, I am become as sounding brass, or a tinkling cymbal.
>
> And though I have the gift of prophecy, and understand all mysteries, and all knowledge; and though I have all faith, so that I could remove mountains, and have not charity, I am nothing.

"Kings and Queens"

"No," he continues, "we can't just treat our patients medically. We have to treat them as individuals, as kings and queens, and we have to maintain their dignity as such, as kings and queens."

And that is why he came to the City of Hope. I asked, "How long have you been here?" His reply came back without a moment's delay: "Ten years and three months." [*Now twenty-one years.*]

Every day in that period has been a revelation and an opportunity to carry out his life's mission. "Here we are free to use our skills and we can't help but love our work. We are not selling health on the hoof; we are preserving human identity, the selfhood of the individual. That patient is never just a sick thumb; he is a whole person; he's not just a physical body, he's a spiritual being.

"Or consider that man lying in a bed that costs $30,000 a year to maintain. We have no right to burden him with the cost; he has enough burdens already. He has come to us with three questions: 'Can I be cured? Will I suffer great pain? Will I be abandoned?' And the most important question for him is the last one.

"It is the key question *we* must answer, and from the moment he arrives we let him know that we will be by his side. Whatever happens, he will not be isolated in a death wing just to make things more convenient for doctors and nurses. Even when a patient becomes terminal you can still give something—a little of yourself."

Happily, surgery can do much for many cancer patients, and nothing so thrills a surgeon as sending someone back into the bosom of his family to lead a normal life again. Sometimes the physician must make his compromise and offer an amputation on the altar of the disease. Among Dr. Byron's greatest satisfactions are the procedures he has developed to reduce deformities resulting from surgery, to obviate blood losses, to reduce the time spent on the operating table, and to simplify procedures for his fellow-surgeons.

The policy at the City of Hope is to play for every advantage on the patient's behalf. Except in emergencies, Dr. Byron allows a week before surgery during which the patient is helped to mobilize his psychological and spiritual defenses. Studies conducted at the City of Hope indicate that this practice hastens recovery and adjustment.

Spirit of Renewal

Dr. Byron is involved in all three aspects of City of Hope work—patient care, research and teaching. He is hard-pressed to say which has greater fascination for him. In cancer seminars he is much sought after by his fellow-professionals; his articles and papers are widely circulated in the professional journals; films that he has prepared on surgical techniques are used in the medical schools and in the societies concerned with oncology.

But there is a special exhilaration in his voice when he speaks of the educational work he has directed at the City of Hope. He prefaces an explanation of his attitude with a passage from Deuteronomy: "Thou shalt love the Lord thy God with all thy heart and with all thy soul and with all thy might. And these words, which I command thee this day shall be upón thy heart. Thou shalt teach them diligently unto thy children, and shalt speak of them when thou sittest in thy house, when thou walkest by the way, when thou liest down, and when thou risest up. Thou shalt bind them for a sign upon thy hand, and they shall be for frontlets between thine eyes. Thou shalt write them upon the doorposts of thy house and upon thy gates: That ye may remember and do all my commandments and be holy unto your God."

As he sees it, the mandate is to learn the healing ways of love and to teach them diligently. It is incumbent on him to share his knowledge with others so that human kindness may be spread in an ever-widening orbit. He speaks with pride of the sixty young men whom he trained personally in surgery at the City of Hope during the past ten years; some spent six months with him, others as much as two years. He keeps track of them. Once a year, those who are within reach of Dr. Byron's home assemble with their families on his lawn for a barbecue at which they exchange informally the news about their work. Some of his students are now saving lives in Africa, India and Okinawa. Twelve of them are professors in medical schools.

The cancer cells against which he wields the knife are killers because they have a terrible capacity to multiply themselves. When the good and wholesome in mankind can multiply itself with equal success and can be mobilized for the fight, the victory will be won. Meanwhile Ralph Byron renews himself in the young people he sends forth from the City of Hope to light their candles in the dark places of the world.

His preoccupations have made Dr. Byron a serious, even solemn person as he confronts the challenges of a daily struggle with death. Periodically he pauses to allow his humor to come to the surface. His lectures, though filled with Biblical and literary allusions to emphasize a point, nevertheless have room for stories, of which this is a sample: A nine-year old was asked by his teacher to write a composition telling all about himself. He asked his mother where he came from and received the conventional reply, "The stork brought you." And daddy? Same answer. And grandpa? The stork brought him too. The next day the boy turned in his essay, which began with this sentence: "At the outset of this composition I would like you to know that there hasn't been a normal birth in our family for the last three generations."

I asked Dr. Byron the reason for the City of Hope's high reputation. He offered two factors. First, he said, is the close link between the clinician engaged in medical treatment and the researcher working in the laboratories of the Medical Center. "We work as a team; our departments are not isolated from each other." The second reason, he continued, is this, "The secret of success is to know your objective and never lose sight of it."

That has been a maxim observed by the City of Hope: the objective is always, and unswervingly, the patient. And it has been observed by Dr. Byron in his own life. From his youth he knew exactly what his goal would be. He had known it ever since the day he read in the Book of Ezekiel: "And I sought for a man among them, that should make up the hedge, and stand in the gap before me for the land, that I should not destroy it: but I found none."

He knew that so long as a gap existed between life and death, he would have to be a man in the hedge.

17 They Call Him Doc

In the world of medicine he is Ralph L. Byron, Jr., M.D., F.A.C.S. But to a host of men and women, numbering in the thousands, he is Doc.

They are the King's Couples Class of the Lake Avenue Congregational Church in Pasadena, California, a group he has taught for years and their aggregate membership now approximately totals six thousand. Currently the membership is 136 couples plus ten or twelve members who are not coupled. They represent practically every profession, and like their teacher, give evidence of being a highly motivated group of men and women.

No book about Ralph Byron would be complete without some contribution from a cross section of his King's Couples. What comes to mind when they think of the dynamic person they call Doc?

The thing I remember most about Dr. Byron is—that he is always willing to listen to any problem anyone has, and that a person can feel free to call him to discuss the problem. He is a great strength in time of need. My wife and I have called on him several occasions during the past ten years that we have known him. He has always been right there.

Good old Doc! He has his own brand of dry humor. I remember one Sunday morning during class in early 1976 he said, with a straight face, "Last week the FBI contacted me about a member of this class. I told them that the class member they were inquiring about wasn't perfect, and that he was the man they were after."

Even though my wife and I knew what Doc was referring to, we realized by the expressions on some faces that others didn't know what he was talking about. We slid down in our seats slowly as some had to think that the FBI was looking for a criminal suspect in our class, when in fact I was in law enforcement for twelve years and had been nominated to attend the national FBI Academy. I had used Doc as a personal reference on the application. Thanks to Doc and others, I was finally selected to attend.

The thing I will never forget about Dr. Byron is—the time at Alpine Lodge at a King's Couples Retreat in the mountains, I forgot my medicine, and had a bad asthma attack. At 1:00 A.M. Doc drove down the mountains to San Bernardino to the hospital and brought back medicine. He got a pharmacist to go to the hospital in the middle of the night. After returning he then had to go pick up Dorothy in Arcadia at 6:00 that morning.

While president of King's Couples, I had to go to the home of a couple who were having marital problems, where the husband had left. I called Doc at 10:30 P.M. He said, "Shall we go together?" We did. Praise the Lord for Doc.

Even though we are in our forties, Doc and Dorothy are like parents to us. They show real concern, care, and give guidance to us.

When I think of Dr. Byron, I always remember—first meeting him. It was a Saturday afternoon, and we were at a church picnic. As president of the King's Couples Sunday school class, I had been notified that our regular teacher would be absent the following day.

One of the church pastors mentioned to me that Dr. Byron might be available and pointed him out to me since he was new at LACC. I walked up behind Dr. Byron, who was seated at a table having lunch with his family, introduced myself, and then proceeded to explain about our lack of a teacher for the following morning. As I recall, he responded with two questions, "What age group is the class?" and "What time do you meet?" I explained that it was a newly married couples class, and we met at 9:30 A.M. His comment was "I'll be there"—and that ended our conversation. Walking away, somewhat puzzled over this *man of few words,* I returned to my wife and explained that we now had a teacher for the following morning, though admittedly I wasn't sure what kind of a message we would be getting. For those of you who have heard Dr. Byron, the answer to that question would be the same then as it is today. Dr. Byron has the amazing ability to make Scripture *live,* and by his method of repeating verse after verse, a person can't help but learn the verses himself. His fantastic ability to quote Scripture from memory is a challenge to all of us as to how God's Word can be stored in our hearts.

In the course of time and without question according to God's will, Dr. Byron was asked to be the regular teacher of the King's Couples class, which he ultimately accepted. Hundreds or even thousands of people by now can attest to the faithfulness and steadfastness of the Doc in teaching that class along with his multitude of other duties.

I thank the Lord for this man, and only God knows how many thousands have come to Jesus Christ because of him. Praise the Lord!

What kind of person is Dr. Byron?—how can I ever forget Doc's wonderful treatment of my mother? We were humble people. My parents had worked hard all their lives, and my mother had not known what it was to be treated *special.* Then, while she was visiting us from the east, she became very ill, and Doc arranged for her to have the needed surgery at the City of Hope. I was with my mother one day when she was beginning to recover. Dr. Byron came in, checked her over, then said, "I think you're well enough to take a little walk." He then reached down and got her slippers, helped her put them on, took her by the arm, and walked her out to the nearby rose garden. There, he plucked a rose (an unusual occurrence for the roses are for enjoyment by everybody), handed it to her ceremoniously, and walked her back to her room. "I felt like a *queen,*" my mother told me.

That's the kind of person Doc is.

What impresses me most about Dr. Byron is—his *consistent* testimony for Jesus Christ, his consistent time devoted to the Word of God and his uncompromised life, as far as the world is concerned. Yet, *all* are invited to his home on occasions such as the yearly Christmas sing, when many of his Jewish doctor friends congregate there to sing God's praises with those who love Jesus.

As we break bread together, they feel God's love and Doc's great love for them. During Doc's message, he includes many Scriptures from the Old Testament pertaining to "the house of Israel." These same Jews return to Doc's home time and time again, *knowing* that they will hear the Gospel. His memory of the Word of God is tremendous—his source of *power.*

The most unforgettable thing about Dr. Byron is—Doc's testimony as a *Christian* at City of Hope. He is the busiest person I have ever known, and yet he was concerned enough with me, as an individual, to assist in a gallbladder surgery which was performed on me. He adjusted his schedule, just so he could be there at the hospital that particular day. He also operated on my father for cancer.

When we were on a retreat at Alpine Lodge near Lake Arrowhead, Lyle and Lois Grotjohn's daughter, Lonnie, was seriously injured when an automobile ran over her leg. Doc left the conference of his own King's Couples Sunday school class in order to enter Kaiser Hospital to make sure that Lonnie had the best doctor and the best care possible. He has *always* gone beyond the call of duty and beyond his own strength to help others.

What is most outstanding about Dr. Byron is—his life as a family man which is beyond compare. He is the busiest person I've ever met, and still he maintains his *rocking chair* where he sits as the family members share their joys and trials. He takes the *time* for the most important things that *God* gives him to do. He provides for his family *spiritually.* He seems to be a great husband and father. He maintains a sense of humor, even though he is tired. His supernatural strength is gained through Bible reading and prayer, and he gives all the glory to God!

I understand that Doc has loaned money to those involved in unsuccessful business dealings, and has always given of himself to *up* and outers as well as to down and outers. He is *God's* man of the hour.

The thing that continually amazes my husband and me is—Dr. Byron's utter dependability. We've been in King's Couples about fourteen years and it's unbelievable how few times he has missed. Even with his time-consuming traveling, he has such a commitment to our class that he somehow manages to be back for Sunday morning. Sometimes he has to scoot right out afterward to fulfill an engagement; sometimes he has already been speaking to a group, or, as an example, on City of Hope Sunday, he is at the radio station in Los Angeles for a live broadcast at 7:30 in the morning. (Once a year, in the manner of the Heart Fund or the March of Dimes, the City of Hope receives support from the general public.)

And Doc is a car nut. You should just see his car. No matter what kind it is, it's shining like nobody else's. Dorothy says he never washes his car; he uses Pledge wax—cans and cans of Pledge. Even when he comes home after hours in surgery, he's out there in his bare feet shining his car. That's Doc. He does nothing by halves!

The testimony I can give to Dr. Byron is— the influence he has had on my life. My mother, a Christian woman, had been left by my father to bring up her children alone. She had to work to support my brother and me. Somehow she became involved in an investment affair which proved fraudulent. Although she was in no way responsible, Mother was convicted and sent to prison. She didn't complain or become bitter against God. She actually witnessed of her faith in Christ while in prison. But she became ill and was placed in the prison hospital. It got so I just couldn't bear it! My mother—sixty years old—sick in that prison. I decided to tell Doc. We went to the house and blurted out the whole story to Doc and Dorothy. It was so embarrassing. Me—a Christian and a member of the King's Couples class—and my mother a convicted prisoner!

I'll never forget how they took it. They listened, then Doc said very softly, "But for the grace of God I might have been the one in prison." Then I shared with him that my mother would never do the thing she was accused of doing. Once when she was working for a businessman, he said, "Tell whoever calls that I'm not in." Mom wouldn't stoop to such a lie. "Tell him yourself," she answered.

Dr. Byron got into action, and soon mother was moved to the City of Hope. There too she was a great witness to the staff.

We will always feel greatly indebted to our teacher, Doc.

What can I tell you about my teacher, Doc Byron?—I can never forget Doc's total commitment to me and my family. He is the primary one who puts flesh and bones on the words *faithfulness, loyalty,* and *availability* for me. His generosity and willingness to go the second mile have stunned me on more than one occasion.

No book about Doc would be complete without making the readers aware that he is a *football fanatic* (University of Southern California Trojans); also as a golf partner, he's a heckler *par* excellence. Often when I've been faced with a difficult putt, encouraging remarks such as "I'll bet that makes your mouth dry up" would shatter my concentration! (Doc has a putting green in his backyard.)

Doc's ministry has effected terrific changes in my life. Since the shared life of Jesus Christ is what sets us believers apart from the rest of the world, implanted in us, that life has a character and goal of its own, growing up in Christlikeness. The issue for us is how do you teach someone to LIVE? Modeling Christlikeness is the process.

An idea reaches the *mind*. A life reaches a *life*. When I think of *living epistles,* it is Dr. Byron who has modeled for me:

1. Loving my wife as Christ loved the Church
2. Setting aside my personal interest in order to meet the needs of others
3. The highest respect for and absolute trust in the Word of God (cover to cover)
4. Consistent love that is not dependent on my response
5. Dependability which means keeping a promise even if it ruins me
6. Effective, consistent prayer life

I could never repay Doc for his unmerited love shown to me and my family—so I'm asking *God* to!

"I didn't know that being a Christian could be such fun, till I met Doc and Dorothy Byron," a newcomer to the King's Couples commented. And fun it is, for like most organized adult classes, Doc's group programs a balance of recreation into their activities which even include a shish kebab. King's Couples class is fortunate in having a nucleus of warmhearted, sharing Armenian members, and for some years they have spearheaded (if you'll pardon the pun) a spectacular dinner held at the Byron home. They can count on about 350 being present on the attractive grounds which Doc himself spruces up for the occasion.

Viewing the quantities of lamb sizzling over the red coals on the ingenious, motor-driven skewers, a first-timer facetiously queried the host "Are you starting your own Day of Atonement, Doctor?" Following the feast, which is complete with Armenian dessert goodies, there is a sing. One time one of the numbers led by opera singer Chris Lacona (a K.C. member) was "Old Doc Byron Had a Farm." When the group came to the lines, "with a quack-quack here and a quack-quack there . . . ," Chris halted the song to ask "Hey, what's *Doc* doing with a quack?"

There's more than food and fun. For Dr. Byron never forgets that in every King's Couples crowd are some people who do not know Jesus as Savior and Lord. So in a brief, interesting, and punchy message, he offers them an opportunity. Among them are sure to be some of his own colleagues and associates from the City of Hope.

But Doc is not the only one who invites unsaved colleagues and friends. Nearly every Sunday, quite a number of newcomers come to the class from both nearby and some distance. Why do class members unhesitatingly invite friends and neighbors to their Sunday school class? Here are some of the reasons they have shared:

> I can always feel confident about inviting an unsaved friend; I know he'll get something for his mind as well as his heart.

> There's something about Doc that always makes Christianity look good. When I've brought someone to class, I've found it's been easier to witness to him afterward. People appear to be more open to listen after they have heard Doc expound the Bible.

A class gets like its teacher; King's Couples exudes enthusiasm.

Ours is more than a Sunday school class. It's a loving family. When one of us is ill or in trouble, our Heart Line goes into action immediately. We start a chain of continual prayer. Not only that, but we move in with practical help, providing the meals, caring for the children—whatever is most needed, is lovingly done. Maybe, through the years this has been a matter of our teacher's motto, *Standing in the gap*, rubbing off on the rest of us.

Some people who know Dr. Byron have asked whether it makes any difference to the class being taught, when the teacher not only knows the Bible but is something of an authority on the chemistry of the human body? The answer is an unqualified yes, and perhaps one of the best examples would be excerpts from one Sunday's lesson.

The text was the ninth chapter of Hebrews. Perhaps we need to add that in the King's Couples class, the reading of the Word of God has high priority. It's never a casual part. In the same way that someone is responsible each week for the praying, the music, and announcements, so is it prearranged who will read the Scripture. This allows for it to be read well and meaningfully before the teacher begins his exposition. On this particular Sunday, blood was the prominent theme of the text. At one point Dr. Byron screwed up his face, shook his head, and said, "Blood. Such an offensive thing to talk about!" Then in a characteristic, half-joking twist of his mouth, he countered his own argument with "Not in heart surgery; nothing offensive about blood there." This led to his ready reciting of "the life of the flesh is in the blood" (Leviticus 17:11), and he, the surgeon now, was off—on a favorite topic.

" 'The life of the flesh is in the blood.' This astonishing statement was made thirty-five hundred years ago when the blood and its circulation were little more than a mystery. It was not for another thirty-three hundred years that William Harvey described the circulation of the blood through arteries, into the capillaries, and back to the heart through the veins. However, in the last two centuries the significance of this statement has grown as we have come to realize the multitude of life-giving properties in the blood.

"The basic fluid in the blood is water. Because of its specific heat, water is great for regulating temperature. We think our cars are good if they don't boil over going up the mountains. However, the engine temperature may go from fifty degrees to 205 degrees. In contrast, our bodies maintain a very constant temperature, ninety-eight to ninety-nine degrees whether we are walking, climbing, or sitting. Our body could not survive if the temperature were to rise much over 110 degrees. The color of the blood, red, results from the presence of hemoglobin. This protein has the ability to pick up oxygen at the lungs and give it off at the cell, and all at body temperature. And it does it efficiently. Now there are many substances that will either pick up oxygen or give it off. Hemoglobin does both. Oh, you say, since it's so valuable, I would like you to inject hemoglobin into my bloodstream. Alas! It would clog your kidneys and perhaps take your life. The hemoglobin must be in a nice envelope—the red cell. The cell membrane permits the oxygen to pass in and out with ease, but it holds the hemoglobin in. God was mindful of this when He made us.

"A friend of mine took the various properties such a cell would need to have, and he programmed this into a sophisticated computer. On the oscilloscope flashed the ideal shape—a biconcave disk which just happens to be the shape of the red cell!

"The body can be likened to a great fortification, where the white blood cells are the soldiers. These polymorphonuclear cells are important in fighting infection. Without them a person becomes prey to every bacterial infection that passes by.

"There is evidence that thirty-two *T* lymphocytes can destroy one cancer cell. The platelets are the thumb in the dike, without which we would bleed into the tissues and from the nose and mouth. The globulin is important for immunity, and the albumin which keeps us from getting edema (dropsy) is vital or we would swell up like a balloon. Without the fibrinogens, significant in clotting, it would be difficult to stop bleeding, even from a small cut."

No class of medical students was more intent as Doc continued.

"In the blood are various electrolytes—sodium, potassium, chloride, and others. The amount of each is quite constant. Thus sodium is normally about 135 milliequivalent. If it drops below 110, the person's life is in jeopardy. The blood carries amino acids, glucose, and lipids to the cells, and dispatches waste products also. In the blood are minute amounts of hormones such as thyroglobulin. Without it we become slow, sluggish, and inactive. If there is too much we become hyperactive, nervous, jittery individuals."

The question was raised What of the person who will not accept a blood transfusion? Dr. Byron explained the policy at City of Hope.

"It used to be that we would not accept such persons as patients at the City of Hope. After all, no one likes to lose. We surgeons play for keeps. We reversed this policy, however. We figured the patient would likely go somewhere else, perhaps to a place where they perform the particular needed operation about once in five years. With our experience in doing the same surgery a hundred or so times a year, we would have that much more chance of pulling him through. Moreover, at City of Hope our creed is 'You have a need; we will help you meet it.' We operated on one *no blood* patient and he survived. But later when he was bleeding from a duodenal ulcer he insisted, 'I would rather *die* than accept a blood transfusion.' He got his wish.

"Yes, the blood is most remarkable in its makeup, critical balance, and function. Like a small stream, the blood is introduced in Genesis, pictured in the law by the sacrifices, and finally comes, like a mighty river, to fruition and fulfillment at the cross. 'Neither by the blood of goats and calves, but by his own blood he entered in once into the holy place, having obtained eternal redemption for us' (Hebrews 9:12). 'Without shedding of blood is no remission' (Hebrews 9:22). 'And, having made peace through the blood of his cross, by him to reconcile all things unto himself' (Colossians 1:20)."

Rarely does a session close after such a presentation without someone making a decision to accept Christ or to commit his life more fully to God.

18 That's My Dad!

It's true that certain characteristics, traits, and quirks will never be as clearly delineated as when they are expressed by the family of the person concerned.

We have a rare opportunity to listen in as the four Byron children tell who Ralph Byron, the surgeon, is as their *father*. The occasion was the Sweetheart Banquet of the King's Couples class in February 1976 when they honored their teacher with a *This Is Your Life, Doc* celebration. This was a total surprise to Dr. Byron: the class collaborators had invited him to be the speaker and the program bore this out. At the appointed time the minister, Dr. Ortlund, took over in his uninhibited fashion. Predictably, many tributes were paid by friends, old and new, and by professional colleagues. But the most hilarious moments were when the four Byrons—Joanne, Rod, Jon, and Rick—shared, what to them is, the essence of their Dad.

Sparkly Joanne, as the eldest Byron, was first to speak.

Well—let's see. My Dad and Mom have been *fantastic*. Dad has always been the same; you could always count on him to react the same. If you knew you had done something wrong, you could be sure he would act the same. There was never anger. When he made a strange face, you knew he was upset.

When I was in high school and wasn't doing well, he told me he would get up every morning and study chemistry with me. He did, though this meant he had to get up even earlier for his own Bible study. He drove me to school from the time I was in junior high all through high school. Every day he lectured me on how I could get better grades, and the entire time that we would drive, I would put my makeup on. I just turned him off. I didn't even *hear* what he said. It was the same, morning after morning; I would get in the car, and Dad would start in—it was like an instant replay. But I just clicked it off. When we would get to school, I'd get out and say "see you tonight," and he'd wave bye and drive off. Then one day I said, "Dad, you know I never hear what you say morning after morning." "That's all right," he answered, "I'll just keep saying it." And he did. That's my dad. He's not a quitter; he always looks at things optimistically, always believes something good is going to come out of everything.

Sometimes he attempts what is very obviously the impossible. We had a gigantic oak tree in our yard, and one morning after a bad windstorm I ran in the house and said, "The tree's falling on the house." Dad scratched his head and grunted, "Well, well, well—the tree—well, well." He just kept saying that, then he said, "Well—I'll be back." He stepped to the garage and came out with a saw in his hand, a regular, ordinary handsaw. Then he started on the oak tree! I remember saying to Mom, "He's never going to get through it." And my wise mother said, "Leave him *alone;* you can't talk to him when he's like this, leave him alone." I called Bill (it was just before we were married), and when he came over, he eyed the situation and concluded, "You're not gonna do it, Doc."

"I need an *axe,*" Dad muttered. Ultimately we had to call a tree removal company, but not before Dad had exhausted all the possibilities. That's my Dad!

As a fellow surgeon, as well as a son-in-law, Dr. Bill Northrup (Joanne's husband) added:

When my wife and I came to the City of Hope for a year, it was as much to be with Ralph as to have a great experience in surgery. And it's been more than I expected. I should say that I didn't start out as a Ralph Byron fan. I had wondered if some of the things I had heard about him—his dedication and all—were not a little larger than life! Then I got to know him. One thing that is so *super* about my father-in-law is that he views life as a contest and that he is a contestant who will always win in any encounter he has. His optimism, his enthusiasm in everything and with everybody, is unparalleled. I've never met anybody who had his firm conviction that he will win in whatever he gets involved in. And he truly enjoys everything. He gets a kick out it. Sometimes we laugh till we cry. Ralph can be hilarious, and it's good for all of us. I have learned that he's for real, that all his optimism and what he says are not part of a put-on—not the repertoire of Dr. Ralph Byron. I tend to be up and down; so his approach to life has been good for me. He really is smelling roses and picking daisies every minute, and enjoying it.

Next in line is number one son, Rod, and his wife, Doris. Rod is well along in his medical studies, and his sharp and pretty wife is a news reporter and journalist. Rod shares his perception of his Dad.

Well, my Dad is a very special person to me. Where to begin? Just let me say a couple of things are really, *really* important to my Dad. Number one, he gets up early in the morning—you know, six o'clock or earlier. Me? I always hated to get up in the morning. But once in a while I would, and there Dad would be in his rocking chair with a cup of coffee nearby. He'd be leaning back in that old rocker with his feet up on the kitchen counter and he'd be dressed in his underwear and his old bathrobe. He would have his Bible out and he would be reading it and praying. You couldn't be quite sure if he was asleep or not; you had to have faith that he was not. After this—I don't know if it's that he doesn't do his best praying in the house—he would go outside. Now in the winter it can be pretty cold out there and you really have to picture this. (When I was young I never wanted any of my friends to come over at this time.) Running around with the lawnmower would be Dad with his bathrobe knotted in the middle and flapping. It was the funniest thing; the lawnmower would be going much too fast, but this was Dad's attempt to make his golf course grass grow. "Just give me a couple of weeks and we'll have it green," he would say. It was just *weeds*. But his persistence paid off.

What I'm saying—why these two things are important to me—is that I learned something from this; I learned that you really must stick with things. You can go out there now (everybody knows my Dad's golf course), and give him credit. It's pretty good! So I learned the value of persistence. Through my Dad's morning after morning, year after year, keeping of his appointment with God—letting nothing interfere with it—I learned about consistency. That's my Dad!

Next come Jon and his Francie (who accepted Christ at the King's Couples). Jon draws himself up to his tall height and quips, "I'm the one Byron who can look down on my Dad; I'm the only one over five feet ten inches!"

My Dad and I during the past year have gone into a little business venture together: we did an album together. No, he didn't sing on the album; I did. But Dad was the financial backer for this venture, and it was a great experience for me. Because of that, my Dad and I have grown very close as we've had experiences together. When I first broached the idea to him, we were talking in terms of a sum between three and four figures, nearer to four. It was rather exciting, everybody was happy about the idea, and Dad had settled in his mind that it was going to cost this much. Then, as I began to talk with other people, they kept telling me how neat it is if you can get other special effects in your album. I thought, *Oh boy, that would be a lot of fun!* So I did some estimating and came up with a new figure and took this new piece of information to my dad. Well, as Joanne mentioned, Dad has one response to bad news: it's not that he gets angry but he whistles. Not whistling really; it's more like blowing hot air out of his mouth. I should have kept this in mind. We have a saying in our house: "Dad is not good at surprises." He will tell you this himself. He admits that he doesn't trust his own first reaction to something thrown at him unexpectedly. It's after he has had his time with the Lord, and he has sorted out this new whatever-it-is in the quiet of his morning time, that he can give better responses.

But I had just blurted out this new figure for our album. His response? He *whistled*. Finally though, we resolved the problem of the album. He decided I was out of my mind, but after a while, he got into the act, going into it whole hog, and he was enjoying it too. In a couple of weeks our little business venture will come to an end. So tonight I mentioned to him that I was thinking about doing another album. He didn't get too excited about that! But that's Dad!

Rick, you step up to the mike now. Rick is just entering college.

My Dad? My Dad is a unique character. He's a character to me because—well, I don't know how to explain it—but the time he has spent with me was not out of a sense of duty, but was of *love*. He's really made the effort to be a father to me, a teacher to me—all sorts of things. By just letting me absorb the kind of person that he is, in this way I've developed a unique respect for him, and it's really been neat just to grow up with him as my father and to see how he copes with failure and all.

I have a funny story about him: You know, Dad always polishes his car—rubs and shines it. This is usually in the morning. Sometimes he gets involved, and suddenly it'll dawn on him that he has to go to work. Well this happened one morning; there he was in his old bathrobe, shining away at his car. He was going to be late, so he dashed into the house, grabbed his wallet, grabbed his keys, and just as he was hopping into the car, my mother came over and said, "Aren't you going to put something on?"

You see, Dad has a one-track mind.

In all the hilarity of the evening, no one laughed more than the guest of honor. It didn't matter that most of the jokes were on him. And this is one more thing that all four Byrons say of their dad: "He laughs at himself."

The willingness to change is another trait the family attributes to their father. When he's wrong or has made a mistake, he recognizes that he has, and does something about it.

Joanne probably summed up all their feelings when after speaking about her father, she said warmly, "He's the *best*."

19 Witnessing to the Critically Ill

How do you witness to the critically ill? This is a question that comes to me very frequently as a physician and a Christian. It's humbling as well as gratifying to me to know that people expect I am doing this. If I would ever be tempted to curtail my witness—I pray this might never be so—this trust in me would strongly challenge and reinforce me.

I have three prayers as I think of this vital ministry. One, that I might earn the right to a hearing by the patient. There's no law or principle that decrees, just because I'm the physician or surgeon, that the sick person must listen to my views on religion. Not at all! No patient should ever feel he or she has to show some kind of gratitude to the doctor by taking an interest in what he believes. This is what I mean when I say I must *earn the right* to be listened to.

I can't, nor would I dictate, how others should earn this right. For me, it's a matter of being sincerely interested in the patient *as a person.* I can demonstrate this in a number of little ways; how I speak to him, just by a smile, taking a minute to notice him especially, as I would otherwise walk by. Then too, there is the matter of reputation; one patient tells another. The word gets around that I don't badger a person, but rather share and offer him something that's mighty important to me.

My second prayer is that I give the Gospel so clearly that the person could never stand before the Lord and say "I didn't hear." By clear, I have in mind, keeping it simple. So often we tend to make spiritual conversion more difficult than God Himself makes it. I'm reminded that when the Apostle Paul was asked by a desperate man, "What must I do to be saved?" Paul's answer was just one sentence. "Believe on the Lord Jesus Christ, and thou shalt be saved" (Acts 16:30, 31). There's a time to teach the Bible, to instill doctrine, to exhort people to grow in Christ. But when the person is sick and suffering—perhaps dying—all he needs is help to take that one step of faith. The Lord will do the rest.

Thirdly, my prayer is that I will have such wisdom that my witness will not make it difficult or impossible for those who follow. If I am not the one whom the Holy Spirit uses to win a man or woman to Jesus Christ, I pray I will leave the door open for the next Christian witness.

We've all met believers who are zealous, who love the Lord, but who have a bull-in-a-china-shop approach. Common sense should be a major factor in witnessing.

The City of Hope has some ninety-two acres. It would be possible for me to go down to the cafeteria or stand on a curb, and proclaim the Gospel! There might or might not be one or two decisions. However, in about twenty-four hours I would be relieved of my position as chief of surgery, and my opportunity to witness to both patients and staff would come to an abrupt end. But, in a less direct approach, it is possible to get the message out in an acceptable fashion. Here is one example. (It doesn't have to do with witnessing to the sick, but it has a direct bearing on my opportunities at the City of Hope.) The president of the City of Hope wrote me and asked, "Do you think that if Samson were alive today, God could use him?" The implication appeared to be that Samson was not telling the truth, not keeping his vows, and running around with the godless Philistines.

I couldn't know what was behind the question. I wrote the president back and said, "You get your friends together, and in six sessions I will brief you on the Bible from Genesis to Revelation, with no holds barred. I will speak an hour and you may ask questions for an hour." Then began one of the most unusual Bible classes! Thirty-five wealthy members of the Jewish community gathered to study the Bible. They had asked for it, and in return got to hear the Gospel many times each evening! Their comment at the conclusion of the series was "You'll never know how much this has meant to us."

I can only hope and pray that the day will come—and events are indicating that it could be very soon—when my Jewish colleagues, those I work with and so highly regard for their skills and their compassion and dedication, will come to realize *That's what Dr. Byron has been telling us all these years.* And they will have opened eyes and obtained a degree of knowledge which will help them to discern that their Messiah is none other than our Lord Jesus Christ. Meanwhile, I thank God daily that the door is still open to me—after these twenty-two years—to witness to the critically ill, among others.

When we are asked to counsel or speak with the critically ill, it is difficult—very difficult. Why? Often there is nothing that we physically can do for them. This frustrates us, and we transfer their problems to ourselves. Visiting such a person drains us. It means giving our time, our effort, our understanding, a word of comfort, an answered question, or perhaps just being a sounding board, someone they can talk to.

Knowing how difficult it is to make ourselves go to see a critically ill individual, we must be in prayer: "Lord, help me to *want* to go; help me not to show my frustration or lack of enthusiasm; help me to have wisdom in knowing what to do; help me to have the right timing; help me to have the right words to say; help me not to lose sight of the objective, not only to be of general support, but of real spiritual help." Here, more than anywhere else, we need God's leading second by second. Although we may be reluctant or hesitant to go, these are the people who need us the most!

The secret of spiritual power in my own life is the hour I spend each morning with the Lord. It has never been easy for me to get up; in fact it is still difficult every morning. However it pays off; the blessing is super and continues to flood my life. I have a prayer list of subjects I want to be certain to pray for. I periodically tear up the list as answers pour in. With the events of the day particularly in mind, I pray with an emphasis on (1) being available, (2) having wisdom in all my dealings with people and situations, and (3) letting God use me to meet the needs of those around me.

It is hard for our finite minds to grasp the greatness and the power of prayer that is the Christian's heritage. An Aladdin's lamp fades to nothingness in comparison. The instructions and promises are crystal clear. Prayer is ours for the using. As we pray in the name of the Lord Jesus, we are instantly in contact with the God of the universe, the God who is all-powerful, the God who loves us.

The commands are simple: "Ask, and it shall be given you" (Luke 11:9); "Pray without ceasing" (1 Thessalonians 5:17); "Be . . . instant in prayer" (Romans 12:12); "Whatsoever ye shall ask in my name [Jesus], that I will do . . . If ye shall ask any thing in my name, I will do it" (John 14:13–14). There are several conditions that we are to meet. "If ye abide in me, and my words abide in you, ye shall ask what ye will, and it shall be done" (John 15:7). Obviously, it goes without saying, that we can only pray in the name of Jesus, if we know Him.

Praying with the critically ill is of enormous value. Although it is sometimes thought of as a very emotional act, it need not be. The administration of the City of Hope feels that a doctor praying with his patient is too emotional and have forbidden it. However, they are delighted to have Scriptures quoted to a patient! If a patient asks me to pray for him, I tell him that I will in my own prayer time with the Lord. I count it a privilege to do this. It is not necessary to shout or generally make a nuisance of oneself as one prays for the patient. We are not heard because of the loudness of our prayer.

How does one start in hospitals where this is permitted? Sometimes the sick person requests that we pray for him. I will initiate the subject with the question, "Would you like me to pray for you?" People are not offended by such a question, but rather look forward to the prayer and are most appreciative. For some it is the very first time they hear their own name mentioned before God and their special problems made important to Him, who is the Great Physician.

When you pray with a critically ill patient, he senses whether prayer is a dominant part of your life or just a peripheral unimportant practice performed when it is expedient. As you listen to and speak with the friend, you may quietly ask "Have you ever invited the Lord Jesus to come into your life?" If he says no, it is then quite natural to follow with the question, "Would you like to now?" If he says yes, then you will not only help him to pray but will pray for him. Alfred Tennyson put it well, "More things are wrought by prayer Than this world dreams of."

Sometimes the person will express doubt as to whether he has ever accepted Jesus as his Savior. I find that what gave assurance to a young marine back in 1944 is just as effective for my patients at the City of Hope. This young corpsman said he wasn't sure, and it troubled him that he might not be saved. I talked with him, and showed him some verses in the Bible including:

> He that heareth my word, and believeth on him that sent me, hath everlasting life, and shall not come into condemnation; but is passed from death unto life.
>
> John 5:24

Then I suggested, "This is November 24, 1944. Make your decision now, and if anyone ever asks you, you can tell him." We prayed together. He did make his personal commitment to Christ, and his doubts were dispelled, replaced with the peace of God "which passeth all understanding" (Philippians 4:7). The same definite transaction works for the critically ill patient.

20 Letting the Bible Witness

The Word of God makes bold claims for itself. Let's take any other book: you choose one and I will choose one, each book purporting to be the fountain of all wisdom. At this point it's your book against mine. It is not so with the Holy Scriptures. It is totally unlike any other book ever written.

Some people talk about defending the Bible. The Bible is like a lion; let it out, and it will defend itself, every time. What does the Bible say about itself? Among other things, it says "This is the Word of the Lord." And again and again we read "Thus saith the Lord." Then, the Word of God claims to be "quick, and powerful, and sharper than any twoedged sword, piercing even to the dividing asunder of soul and spirit, and of the joints and marrow, [The latter two are in my area!] and is a discerner of the thoughts and intents of the heart" (Hebrews 4:12). Who or what besides God's eternal Word can make such a claim? Even the most highly trained and skilled professional can go only so far in discerning thoughts in another person's mind.

The Bible is "a lamp unto my feet, and a light unto my path" (Psalms 119:105). The Bible deals with every human emotion, and offers the only lasting peace of heart and mind.

One of the strongest incentives for letting the Word of God witness is that God has specifically declared:

> So shall my word be that goeth forth out of my mouth: it shall not return unto me void, but it shall accomplish that which I please, and it shall prosper in the thing whereto I sent it.
>
> Isaiah 55:11

This means that we must be right with God if He is to speak through us. Somehow God uses His Word through a stumbling, stammering me, far more than through a mighty Shakespearean actor who is godless.

I was invited to be on an interview program on the largest color television station in Milwaukee. The woman who ran the show told me it was beamed to more than a million women who were doing their housework and watching the program. She informed me that I could have only seven minutes as she had a number of other personalities to question.

"Can you limit your answers to seven minutes?" She sounded concerned lest I hadn't grasped what she said the first time.

"Don't worry, I'll stop at seven minutes," I said.

The show got under way. The hostess asked me a lead question concerning the City of Hope. I answered, keeping an eye on the clock in front of me. With three and one-half minutes to go in the same tone of voice, I began to quote from the Bible. At the ninety second mark, I started the thirteenth chapter of 1 Corinthians:

> Though I speak with the tongues of men and of angels, and have not charity, I am become as sounding brass, or a tinkling cymbal . . . .

I finished the chapter,

> And now abideth faith, hope, charity, these three; but the greatest of these is charity,

just as the second hand hit the top. It had been exactly seven minutes!

I turned to the woman to give her program back to her as I promised, on time. She had big tears running down her cheeks; she could not say a word. So, I had the whole half hour!

Today it is considered acceptable, almost stylish, to quote from the Bible. This is particularly true if we do it in a normal voice without fanfare and without editorial comment, unless we are asked for it. It turns out that people love the Bible and love to hear it quoted. They will often say "That's beautiful," or "You don't know how much that has meant to me." If it does lead to a question from the individual, and it frequently does, then the presentation of the Gospel comes across normally and naturally. We have come to our top priority objective by way of a question. But the appetizer has been the Word of God itself.

At times I might have a slight tremor in my voice as I start quoting a verse. *What if I should forget—and goof? What is the person thinking? Does he (she) consider me some kind of a religious nut?* At such times it would be easier to say to myself, I wonder if I should do this at another time?

Everybody who strives to witness for the Lord is assailed at times with such thoughts. It's not God's reputation we're worried about. No, it's our own. I guess nobody likes to look like a fool.

When the Billy Graham Crusade was going on in Anaheim, I received a call asking that I read the Scripture. I agreed to do it. Inasmuch as I knew the passage, I decided to quote it instead of reading it. The evening came, the stadium was packed, and there were ten thousand people on the field. I was called on, went to the podium with a closed Bible, and began to quote the passage. I don't know what it was about that sea of faces watching me, but my voice had a tremor in it. Somebody asked my wife, who was sitting in the audience, "Was your husband scared? Was that why his voice trembled?" Dorothy said, "Oh *no,* it was the wind hitting the microphone." Later, she said, "You weren't scared, were you Ralph?" I said, "Oh *yes,* I was."

When you use the Bible with the sick, its impact depends to a degree on whether you really believe it or not yourself. Every Christian has to decide how much of the Bible he is going to believe. Will he believe the parts he understands? Will he believe the parts he likes? Will he believe the parts he can prove? The alternative is to accept all the Bible by faith, believe it all, enjoy it all, and use it with confidence. I have been privileged to be on panels with seminary professors who know much, much more than I. After the questions are over, they frequently come to me saying "We say the same things you do, quote the same passages, but somehow they really listen when you say them." The reason is simple: I really believe the Bible is the Word of God.

The question sometimes comes to me how can you propagate

Christianity in an institution that is so strongly Jewish? Well, at the City of Hope we have no creed (or color) barriers. I personally, just let the Word of God speak for itself. I don't use a ministerial tone; I don't put quotation marks in my voice; nor do I announce "Now I'm going to quote you some verses from the Bible." I just do it.

As I stop by to see a patient, we'll talk about the tumor or the surgery; let her say what is on her mind at the moment. Then in a conversational tone I'll share a little of the Bible. "Thou shalt love the Lord thy God with all thy heart, and with all thy soul, and . . ." (Mark 12:30; Deuteronomy 6:5).

"That's from the *Bible*," the person will interrupt to tell me.

Or I'll be saying "The Lord is my shepherd; I shall not want. He maketh me to lie down in green pastures: he leadeth me beside the still waters" (Psalms 23:1–2), when the patient's face will light up, and he'll say, "I learned that as a boy back home" or "My Dad taught me to say that psalm."

Sometimes I'll idly pick up a Bible on the nightstand or booklet some visitor may have left for the patient. I'll casually read from it or quote verses in it. Almost certainly the patient will then show an eagerness to read it—"Is *that* in there?"—whereas it may have lain untouched and been of no help. There are endless ways in which we can let the Bible speak for itself and do its own witnessing. Generally, the person shows pleasure that he has been listening to something from God's Word. Should we be surprised at this?

I've noticed something that always tickles me when many of our patients come back for their periodic checkup. I ask the patient how he is doing, check the status of his treatment or surgery, and we have a little chat. Then I say, "See you next time" and turn to leave when the patient will call after me, "Hey, Doctor, didn't you forget something?" The patient sounds *so* let down. Then I share a few verses of the Bible with him, and off he goes, satisfied.

21 Witnessing—the Moment of Crisis

I was standing at a washing trough attempting to wash my dungarees (new ones are very difficult to hand wash), and I was singing portions of several songs, none of which I knew more than the first two lines! Without any warning, the officer across from me asked, "What makes you so happy?" I was totally caught by surprise. I blurted out, "I guess I'm just healthy!" What a disaster. Here was a young man to whom I had wished to witness. The opportunity had come and gone with dramatic suddenness. I had blown it. In this instance I would not have a second chance. What had gone wrong? I did a postmortem analysis.

Although I was a born-again believer, somehow I had never prepared myself for the sudden opportunity to witness. Given time, I could slowly assemble my thoughts, and tell someone what I believed. However, I had never crystallized my thinking nor framed in words what I believed. I was unprepared to share my faith on a moment's notice.

In surgery, one goes over and over what he must do if there is sudden massive bleeding at the operating table. If one is to save the patient, he must be able to act quickly, smoothly, and the right way. In the fraction of a second after the bleeding starts, one can see the source. One must put a finger on the bleeding vessel, temporarily control it, then set about to improve exposure, get the proper instruments, be sure one has adequate help, and then go to work to permanently control the bleeding. The key is to go over and over the procedure so that in the moment of crisis, the surgeon knows exactly what to do.

As I analyzed my failure to witness, it was apparent that I had never prepared myself for such an opportunity. I was well prepared for the surgical emergency to save a life physically, but I was not disciplined to share the gospel and be used by God to save a soul. What a tragedy this was.

I set out to correct this. I went over and over what I believed. I put it into words. I made sure that it was available on a moment's notice. I asked God to forgive me, and help me never to make that mistake again.

I've found that Christians are not alone in this problem. After a trip overseas, I was heckling one of our state department officials: "I think some of the people you send abroad really do not know what they believe."

He turned to me with fire in his eyes. "It isn't that we want to send people overseas who don't know what they believe," he retorted. "It's that we can't find people who know what they believe."

It is at once apparent, if we are going to counsel the critically ill patient, we must know what we believe. If we are fuzzy in our own beliefs or unsure of ourselves, this comes through loud and clear. While working in the chemistry lab at college I had an unusual opportunity. One of the two most brilliant boys in the department was using the sensitive balance next to me. Our work at the moment was mechanical and permitted us to talk. I asked Darrell if he had ever taken Christ as his personal Savior. He said, "No—but I am interested in exploring it." We talked about the Gospel for a few moments. Sensing the *kill,* I decided to push for a decision. I said, "Do you have an insurance policy?" He said yes.

"Not much chance you'll need it for a while," I countered. To which he replied, "Right."

Now for the clincher. I said, "Even if there is only a 10 percent chance that the Gospel is right, you should take Christ like you took that insurance policy." I can see him yet. He stopped his weighing, turned, and looked hard at me, and with finality in his voice said, "If it isn't 100 percent, I'm not interested."

Again, I had blown the opportunity. Then I considered Peter's words:

> But sanctify the Lord God in your hearts: and be ready always to give an answer to every man that asketh you a reason of the hope that is in you with meekness and fear.
>
> 1 Peter 3:15

The hope, the blessed hope is: it is sure; it is 100 percent; it is absolutely certain; it is the foundation on which we stand.

There is a rule that you cannot take a person farther than you have gone yourself. This suggests that if you are going to be helpful to the dying patient, your life must be squared away with God. Sanctify the Lord God in your hearts; put your faith into action; confess every known sin; allow Jesus to be Lord of your life. Then, God will be able to use you effectively. It is so important to remember that it is only by His grace that any of us are usable.

When I came to Christ, I was truly born again. Some of my bad habits and actions stopped immediately. It's unbelievable but true. However, there were some habits that I rationalized and kept. Before I became a Christian, I loved to tell smutty stories. I probably had the greatest assortment of these jokes of anyone on the campus of ten thousand students. After I came to Christ, I continued to tell these stories, telling myself, "I don't mean any harm by them. I simply enjoy seeing people laugh." One day I had a unique opportunity to witness to one of my Jewish classmates. I told him how wonderful it was to know Christ as my personal Savior. He turned, looked me straight in the eye, and said, "How does a fellow with a filthy mind like yours have nerve enough to talk about God?" I had torpedoed the opportunity.

The Lord taught me a great lesson. From that moment on, I did not tell smutty stories. The Lord is so good. He gave me a replacement instead of a vacuum in my life. He showed me that it is possible to make people laugh even more with clean stories. It is not the smut of a story that makes it funny, it's the unexpected. The skill I had developed in telling bad stories was immediately put to work, but this time it was God's way. Now my story telling became an asset in furthering the Gospel.

I had not done much witnessing to my peers until I went into the armed forces. As an officer, I found it relatively nonthreatening to witness to enlisted men—but I left the officers alone. Why? I guess that down deep inside, I was afraid they would ridicule me or react violently against me. These were the men with whom I would be working closely for the next eighteen months; it was important to me what they thought of me.

Then one day I was sharing with a minister friend the degree of success I was having in witnessing to the enlisted men.

"What about the officers?" he asked incisively.

Rather sheepishly I replied, "I haven't done anything about them."

"You know, Dr. Byron," he explained, "there are many of us who have opportunity to share the Gospel with the GIs, but most of us can't get near the officers."

I heard him loud and clear! From that time on, the officers around me were, for me, a high priority mission field.

Some years later I was privileged to go to Tokyo. I was amazed at my opportunity to share the Gospel with top doctors, scientists, and government officials. Somehow, being a foreigner, I was more acceptable to my peers than I might have been at home. Standing before 150 of the top biologic scientists, I shared some of our research, then the message of the Bible, and finally my own testimony. I closed with the statement, "You've probably wondered why I came to Tokyo." You could see all of the heads instinctively nod yes. I continued, "I didn't come to Tokyo because I didn't have enough to do; I do. I didn't come because I need more reputation; I don't. I've come for one reason, and that is to share Christ with your doctors, your scientists, your professors, and your students!" I sat down. The dean of the scientists rose to his feet and said in perfect English, "We are indeed impressed with your motive for coming to Japan, to help our doctors, our scientists, our professors, and our students."

In analyzing the rather startling success that God gave me in Tokyo—it appeared that there was a simple pattern:

1. Witnessing to one's peers has to have top priority
2. The Christian has to go to the non-Christian
3. The message has to be simple and straight
4. The undertaking has to be saturated with prayer

5. One's reputation has to be on the line for God, and it must be expendable.

Tokyo was not an isolated situation, but in a sense a prototype for sharing the Gospel far and near with one's peers.

While in the marines as I boarded a plane to fly to Guadalcanal, I breathed a prayer, "Lord help me to witness to everyone on this plane." The flight was to be twenty-four hours long. As I surveyed the passengers, I noted that there were twenty-five men—all destined to be commanding officers in their marine units. Wonder of wonders, there was one extra seat. This gave me an opportunity to change seats every hour, and be next to a different officer in order to get the Gospel to him in a personal way. As we reached the island destination, I realized that God had answered my prayer; every man had heard the Gospel.

Often we find ourselves in complete agreement with the Great Commission, but somehow never get under way. We agree: that a world without Christ is without hope; that the command to go into all the world is clear; that we are to be witnesses for Christ; and that we understand the commands and implications. Somehow we just don't get started, especially with our peers.

Many tales are told about the people who come to visit patients in a hospital. The story is told, for instance, of a visitor to a patient in the intensive care unit.

"I know how sick you are; so don't you try to talk. I'll do the talking," the visitor began.

The patient attempted to say something. Again, the hovering visitor explained, "I understand. You're too sick; so don't try to say anything."

The critically ill woman struggled to get some words out but to no avail.

"That's all right," soothed the visitor. "You're very sick, you know."

Finally the patient managed to gasp, "You—you're standing—on my oxygen—hose!"

Funny? Not very—when you are the patient.

Some people are *born* sick visitors; others just do their best. In either case, to be an effective visitor, counselor, friend, it is wise to find out as much as possible that will contribute to a worthwhile visit.

The doctor is a great source of information (if you can just corner him long enough to question him). How sick is the patient you're going to visit? What is his sickness? Is he critical? Is he likely to die soon? If he recovers, will he be relatively normal? How much does he know of his condition? Is it all right for me to talk to him about it? Is what he has, catching? And so on. It's apparent that answers to some or all of these questions will aid greatly in your knowing how to talk during your visit.

A close relative, particularly a wife or a husband, usually has the answers to many of the questions we want to ask. They may have helpful suggestions as to the needs of the sick relative. I don't make many house calls, but recently a man asked me to come and see his wife who was *dying*. I asked, "What is she like?" His only comment was, "She is failing fast." The house was in a poor neighborhood. The husband and daughter were waiting for me at the door. They ushered me into a musty bedroom where an elderly woman was thrashing around in bed. I went over to the bed and felt her pulse. It was strong and booming. I asked her a few questions. There was no response. I could not see even a hint of comprehension. I said a few words to her, patted her on the forehead, and quietly said good-bye. As I left, I said to the relatives, "You have been wonderful to her, and are doing everything that it is possible to do." They smiled weakly. It was apparent that my visit was really more for them than the patient.

The chief thing is to be available and to be sensitive to the situation. For these two qualities, I ask the Lord each morning that I will have them in good supply for the day, to meet each need as it arises.

One of my responsibilities is chairman of the tumor board (a group of specialists who listen to the story of each person, review the findings, and examine the problem patient who has cancer). As chairman, it falls to me to talk to the patient and the relatives, and tell them the recommendations of the board. Often I have a problem because I don't know how much the cancer victim knows or understands about her condition. In one instance, the patient and her relatives were seated. I approached the patient and asked, "How much do you know about yourself?"

"Not much," she answered.

"You do know what your problem is, don't you?" I probed gently.

"Yes," she said unhesitatingly, "I have cancer."

Now I was ready to talk with her. She was honest, open, and had even alerted me as to the term she would like me to use. She proved to be very easy to talk to and most appreciative.

The briefing on the patient's condition frequently includes spiritual pearls which may be helpful. Recently, the person I was about to visit had just received Christ as her Savior. I was alerted to this by a friend standing nearby. This was my cue to encourage the new convert in what she had done and to give her an opportunity to share her testimony. I must say she was young, radiant, and very excited. The Lord had me there to crystallize her belief and encourage her.

Often a relative comes to me and says "I want you to go to see John and lead him to Christ." I tell such a person that I would love to lead John to Christ, but if he is really to be born again, God has to do the miracle. I am available, willing, but can only move as the Lord opens the way. Actually, one sows, another waters, but God gives the increase. Unless the Lord build a house, they that labor, labor in vain (*see* Psalms 127).

On occasion the relatives will alert me to a problem such as "My son had a bad experience in church some time ago. He is very antagonistic to the Gospel." This isn't exactly a word of encouragement to the person asked to witness, but it's certainly helpful in determining which direction the conversation should go—that is, after a few introductory remarks such as "You seem to be feeling better tonight" or "I hear you have great meals here" (what a laugh: the meals are sometimes terrible) or "Do you have anything you would like to talk to me about, any questions?"

On occasion the request to visit a person comes by way of a friend such as "Mary would like to talk to you." Although theoretically this could be about anything, it frequently means that Mary wants to talk about spiritual things. One has to be careful that he doesn't blow this kind of an opportunity. Miss B. was a Jewish girl of twenty-seven years. She had visited my Bible class and had heard the Gospel a number of times. Now she was very sick in the hospital. She sent word that she would like to talk to me. As I was making my way toward her room I saw a sharp young Christian girl. I had what I thought was a great idea. Why not have this girl go and talk with Miss B.? So I arranged this. What happened? My idea backfired. I was the one the patient had asked for; I was the one she wanted to see. The lovely young Christian's visit was totally ineffective in this instance. Unfortunately, it appeared that I was the only one Miss B. would listen to—and I blew it!

As a caller, I am always surprised at how appreciative and pleased the patient and relatives are that I have come. They seem almost surprised that anyone would make the effort and take the time to make such a visit. It is as if one's very presence had been the sermon. Needless to say, it is always easier when one is appreciated!

Working where I do, I am very conscious of the significance of a person's final words. Very important then, in my estimation, are the words of our Lord just before He ascended back to heaven. He said:

> and ye shall be witnesses unto me both in Jerusalem, and in all Judaea, and in Samaria, and unto the uttermost part of the earth.
>
> Acts 1:8

"Ye *shall be* witnesses." That doesn't leave us an option. It's not an elective. And Jerusalem has to be interpreted as *where we are*. Yet, how often do we set our goals for reaching people for Christ off on a far horizon and fail to witness at home?

One of the greatest joys of my life is a young man named Dewey Cass. Here is how I met him. My boy alerted me to a new hamburger place, *The In-and-out Burger*. He said it was good and I should try it. I went up to the window, gave my order, and was waiting when the cook yelled over to me, "Don't I know you?"

Before I could answer, he said, "You're Dr. Byron. You teach the King's Couples." I stammered, "Yes, but how did you know me?" "Oh," he said, "I visited the class last Easter. I even enjoyed what you said."

"How about coming again next Sunday," I suggested.

"Great," he said, "I'll be there."

I looked for Dewey on Sunday but he was not there. I made it a point to have a hamburger the next week. Again I invited him, and again he agreed to come. However, Sunday came and went without his appearing. My invitation the following week brought the same results—no show.

The class's Sweetheart Banquet was coming up Saturday night; so in desperation I invited Dewey. This time he came with his little wife, Barbara. They seemed to enjoy themselves, and to my surprise they came to Sunday school the next day. At the close of the lesson I gave an invitation to any who wished to accept Christ as their Savior. My heart leaped for joy when Dewey's hand went up.

The following week Barbara made her decision. Then her sisters (twins) came and found Christ. They in turn brought Francie, a beautiful little high school girl, and she came to Christ. I didn't know it, but this little girl would one day be my daughter-in-law! We had a regular revival with one after another of Dewey's friends coming to Christ.

Dewey was amazing, a people-oriented young man with a heart for everyone in need. He had a friendly irresistible way with everyone he met. However, his life to that time had been a mess with his personal affairs all fouled up. He had tried what the world had to offer. He had tried religion: a Roman Catholic by background, he had started to embrace Judaism.

Dewey was soundly converted. His life was transformed. But he had a residue of bad habits and problems and a tendency to slip back into some of his old ways. He got together with me several times a week, and we shared the Scripture together. He grew like a weed. Soon he was being discipled by several strong Christians, and he was on the road to a victorious life, dedicated to serving the Savior.

The Lord has blessed the all-out, *go-for-broke* Christian life (as our minister, Dr. Ortlund, puts it). Dewey is using his abilities as co owner and manager of one of the finest Christian book stores I have ever seen, The Christian Corner in Pasadena. There he has ample opportunity to share his faith, and to encourage other Christians by his enthusiasm.

22 What Should I Tell Them?

Through years of experience with every type of patient, I have learned that the ultimate fear of the terminally ill cancer patient is that we will, at some point, abandon him.

What should one tell a patient who has a catastrophic disease and may well be facing death? Even among doctors there are two schools of thought. One group says you should tell little white lies and deny that the patient has cancer or that he may be facing death. They feel that this is the kindest thing to do and in the patient's interest. However, there is a problem. The *little* lies have to keep getting bigger and bigger. Like the Watergate coverup, it becomes more and more difficult. The patient asks, "If my illness is not so serious, why the massive surgery? Why am I getting worse; why do I feel so miserable? Why am I losing so much weight?"

Finally it is apparent that the doctor cannot tell a big enough coverup lie—and the patient has known for some time that he can't trust his doctor to tell the truth. It ends up a disaster.

The second group—*and I am a strong supporter of this persuasion*—feels the thing to do is tell the patient, but do it in the most optimistic way possible. Personally, I generally wait for the patient to bring up the subject of his condition and the possibility of its proving fatal. I've learned that it's important to listen for the word he uses, and to use that same word in discussing his case with him. If he asks, "Do I have cancer, Doctor?" I answer "Yes, you do have cancer." (He will subconsciously use the word he is least afraid of.) Should I switch words and say, "Yes, you have a tumor," he is likely to react, "A *tumor*—oh, that's *awful*." To him, a tumor is much, much worse than cancer. So, to avoid this catastrophe for him, I'm careful to use his own descriptive word.

There is a predictable series of questions the patients rather routinely ask:

1. Do I have cancer?
2. Can it be cured?
3. If it comes back, is there more that can be done?
4. Will I suffer unbearable pain sometime in the future? And, whether it is voiced in one way or another,
5. Will you abandon me at some point?

Here again, honesty is the best approach—in an optimistic vein. The patient needs all the support we can offer him. There are various ways we can do this. For example, I have a patient scheduled for a particular major operation. Today, fortuitously, I ran into a man on whom I had performed the very same surgery nineteen years ago. I can assure my present patient that this other patient is in perfect health nineteen years later.

These are days when many things can be done if the cancer does come back. It is important that the patient be told this. With all the narcotics, tranquilizers, and pain-relieving procedures, we can assure the patient that he will not suffer too much pain. (Pain tolerance studies go on continuously in our research laboratories.)

However, the big apprehension is "Will they abandon me?" The patient lives in terror that somewhere in the progression of the disease, he will be deserted by everyone, and will be all alone. In the opium dens in Hong Kong, there are little cubicles off the main smoking room. When the opium addicts feel that life is not worth living any longer, they go into a cubicle, lie down, and die a slow, lingering death. Nobody cares. No one is interested; they are totally abandoned. But that's Hong Kong, not the City of Hope.

It is our thinking that through our doors enter the most important persons in the world, *our patients*. If the time comes that they are facing death, it means everything to them to know that we have not forgotten them, that there are those who care. How much this means to the grieving family members also. As one woman phrased it, "My husband was dying. We knew he would not live through the night. He needed almost continuous sedation because of the pain; so I inquired if I should get a special nurse in for him. Then the sweet, lovely nurse told me, 'Your husband is my *only* patient tonight.' " It's important to let the patient know that answers are coming in very rapidly; that even though we cannot cure him now, we may have the solution for him in time.

Our present day society is not geared to face death. When a person is confronted with the possibility of dying, it frequently comes as an unexpected shock. We know about the inevitability of death and taxes, but somehow we assume it can't or won't happen to us.

Even some Christians, for all our quoting of Bible verses about "absent in body, but present in spirit" (1 Corinthians 5:3), when confronted with death, shrink in unbelief; sometimes in rebellion against God.

For others, this information about imminent death can be turned into a very positive blessing. My very good friend, Dr. Robert Munger, was called to Oakland to visit his mother who was dying. She was in her nineties and in a rest home. She had had a stroke, but was mentally alert. Bob talked to her, "Mother you know you are about to die." She said, "I know." He said, "Let's pray that the Lord takes you home in time to spend Easter with Dad and the son you lost many years ago." She agreed with a nod of the head, and he prayed for her. She died three days later on Good Friday morning! She spent Easter with her husband and son.

A patient, Mussey Bennett, had advanced cancer and would soon die. Her esophagus was obstructed by a metastasis, and she could no longer eat. I explained to her that without food she would soon die, and that we could prolong her life by a small operation to place a feeding tube in her stomach. She agreed. I rode up the hospital elevator with her. The elevator operator was a sour, unhappy man with a frown on his face. Mussey said to him, "If you knew my *Jesus,* you wouldn't look so miserable." He answered, "wha—wha—what do you mean, lady?" Later, in the operating room, we were working under local anesthesia. We had our head anesthesiologist at the head of the table to alert us if we hurt her too much. Mussey looked up at him and said, "You know why I want to get through this operation?" He said, "No, lady, why?" She answered, "I want a little more time to serve my Jesus." Afterwards this non-Christian doctor came to me and said, "She sure has a great attitude." She went home, and continued her work at the Port of Call, a Christian Service Center she had started. One Sunday several weeks later she gave what was perhaps her greatest message there, then called me and said, "I think I'd better go into the hospital." I arranged it. She walked into her room, put on a gown, climbed into bed, and went home to be with the Lord, victoriously.

Few women in history have been used as much as my very good friend, Henrietta Mears. It is said that there are 450 people on the mission field who came to Christ under her ministry, caught a vision of the world, got their training, and reached the field to carry on a productive spreading of the Gospel. Henrietta had high blood pressure, a bad heart, and sensed that death was near. She spoke for ten minutes to sixteen hundred people gathered at the Forest Home banquet. Her message was this, "I'm often asked, If I had my life to live over what would I do differently; I would trust Christ more." Three days later the Lord took her home in her sleep. This was her coronation speech, "I would trust Christ more."

In contrast, one of the outstanding authors of our day had created his own religion. I helped a surgeon operate on him for what proved to be a cancer of the ureter (the tube that connects the kidney to the bladder). The surgeon said to me, "I don't usually tell patients they have cancer and have only six months to a year to live, but this man has his own religion and is unusually able to face this." He explained to the patient what he had and that death was facing him in the foreseeable future. This brave, stable, well-adjusted, self-made man fell totally apart, gave up, never left the hospital, and died months before his time.

It is interesting that Hamlet, when philosophizing about death, concluded that he didn't know what was on the other side, so he had better stay in this life. Conversely, the Apostle Paul in the letter to Philippi, concluded that it would be much better to be on the other side with the Lord, but because God might have work for him here, he would gladly stay in this life.

It has come to me at times that there is something dreadfully paradoxical about dying in a place named the City of Hope. To the terminal patient, it may even seem a mockery. And certainly we do not like to lose a patient. It's never easy and we doctors feel the weight of failure when death wins.

Nowhere is failure more devastating than in surgery. I develop a very close relationship with my patients, and in many ways, they are part of my family. When one of them develops a severe complication or dies, it represents a failure of monstrous proportions.

On the cold scientific side, surgery is based on statistics. Thus, in cancer of the breast, if it is not treated, there is an 86 percent chance the patient will not survive five years. Those who are alive will be miserable with extensive cancer. If I treat cancer of the breast, there is a 50 percent chance that the patient will be alive and without any evidence of recurrence five years later. Now it is at once apparent that it is highly desirable to treat such a cancer. I know in advance that 50 percent will have developed a recurrence in that same five year period, even though many of them are still alive. I experience a sense of failure when the tumor reappears. In some operations the mortality from the surgery is 5 percent. This simply means that one out of twenty such patients dies. I don't know which one it will be, but when it occurs, I am bombarded with the frustration of failure.

After evaluating the surgery itself, I take a prayerful look at the spiritual aspects of the failure. God knows how I love my work and how much it means to me. He knows that it is an area where He can deal with me.

God has made us so we must come to the Savior by faith. Now if I as a Christian surgeon never had a complication, never had a patient die, and had a 100 percent success rate, it would be apparent that every surgeon should be a Christian. It would not be a matter of faith, but an obvious conclusion. However, it is not possible to prove mathematically that my results are better than those of a non-Christian surgeon. However, they should be just as good as the best. Being a Christian is not a cover-up for being less than the best.

When I fail with a patient, I say, "Thank You, Lord. Do You have lessons for me to learn?" (I always secretly hope that it will be an example of my suffering for righteousness' sake!) However, invariably there are lessons for me to learn, directions that need to be changed, and priorities that have to be reestablished. I immediately begin to make the corrections and adjustments. Again, I breathe a prayer of thanks to the Lord and ask Him to help me not to repeat the same mistakes.

I live in and rest in the promises of God. Like a pilot who has just crashed, I take off again knowing that my God is able to supply all my needs. Failure in surgery is no different from failure in other areas of my life. In each area of failure I follow the surgical rule: "Everyone gets into trouble, but it is the good surgeon who knows how to get out." Hats off to the past; coats off to the future.

We have two kinds of news for our patients—good and bad. Whatever our approach or our philosophy of what we should tell them, good news puts wings on my feet as I carry it to the patient and the relatives.

I have just returned from the operating room. This lady of seventy had, by all our tests, cancer of the large bowel. To make matters worse, the woman's husband, a concert violinist, had died of cancer a few weeks earlier. Lightning was striking twice in this family in rapid succession. A pall of gloom hung over this lady and her family. Then at the operating table, we discovered that the narrowing was not due to cancer and was easily corrected. We were surprised and delighted. You can imagine the response of the family when they heard the good news. They were ecstatic.

Sometimes we focus our attention on the patients who do not do well. In so doing we miss or forget the host of successes that we have. My patients come by referral from other doctors. Not all of these prove to have cancer. (Of course, we cure the ones who don't have a malignancy!)

It's just great to be the bearer of the good news, "You don't have cancer; it's *not* malignant," but unbelievably, some patients seem almost to be disappointed by this good word. They get over this in a hurry as I explain to them that it may be more exciting for me to tell a patient he needs surgery for his cancer, but it is infinitely nicer to not have any cancer that requires treatment. Surgery is good, but only if you need it!

Being a bearer of good news can lead to lots of things. There was Arnie Krueger, an auto racer whose car advertises "R.F.C.—Racers For Christ." Arnie's racing days seemed at an end when he came to the City of Hope. It was my happy privilege to be the one to tell him, "Arnie, you do *not* have cancer." His glad response was to recommit his life to Christ for a new start. "It's not that our organization, Racers For Christ, is trying to push religion at anyone," he explained. "It's just that auto racers have death looking over their shoulders at all times, and you sort of get a closer feeling for God" (From *Los Angeles Herald-Examiner* interview). What a good feeling it was to be able to help him, not only in a physical and a spiritual way, but the Lord spoke to me about backing him financially so he could get going again. You can believe that since then I've had a real interest in auto racing.

Of the patients that truly have cancer, we are able to cure well over 50 percent. These become exciting patients who have won their battle with malignancy. It is great for the patient and exciting for the doctor. All the world loves a winner!

I remember one patient who had made up her own mind. She greeted me with this request: "Doctor, before you take me to surgery, will you please just give me a week to pick out my burial plot?"

"Give you a *week*—buy a cemetery lot! No, I won't. I'll give you just one day to buy a beautiful dress to wear to celebrate when you get out of here."

For the patients in whom the tumor is not curable, there are now a number of chemicals, immunology techniques, and special methods of giving irradiation. This means that there is a series of things which can be done—each with a measure of hope of success. Somewhere on the horizon there is a cloud the size of a man's hand. Elijah knew that this signaled the end of the drought and that a mighty rainstorm was on its way. We, too, see in this small cloud, a rainstorm of better answers to the cancer problem on the way. This results in a great encouragement of hope for the patient under present modes of treatment.

> Hope wakens courage. He who can implant courage in the human soul is the best physician.

Finally, there is the opportunity of being honest with the patient. He learns that he can trust me not only in bad news but in good news. I have learned that the patient fears that he will be abandoned. I am able to assure him that I and the City of Hope will *not abandon* him. And now abideth faith, hope, and love. What a privilege to team these up in caring for a patient.

Ultimately, whether, as doctors, we succeed or fail, "it is appointed unto men once to die" (Hebrews 9:27). As has been said, we come into this world the victims of a terminal disease, the universal sickness, *sin*. But thanks be to God there is a sure cure. We're not dependent upon the latest research; we are not awaiting the newest discoveries to cure this malady of sin. No, for *Christ Jesus came into the world to save sinners*.

Nothing we can tell the victim of a catastrophic disease—not the promise of new treatment—not the hope of a bright tomorrow when a cure will surely be found—not the assurance his pain will be alleviated: none of this can hold out for him the hope and the peace that is found in trusting Jesus Christ. For the believer in Him, there is an eternal tomorrow.

> And God shall wipe away all tears from their eyes; and there shall be no more death, neither sorrow, nor crying, neither shall there be any more pain . . . .
>
> Revelation 21:4

This is the message entrusted to the Christian surgeon, the surgeon of hope.